Social Psychological Approaches to Health

Social Psychological Approaches to Health

Derek R. Rutter
Lyn Quine
David J. Chesham

Centre for Research in Health Behaviour
Institute of Social and Applied Psychology
University of Kent at Canterbury

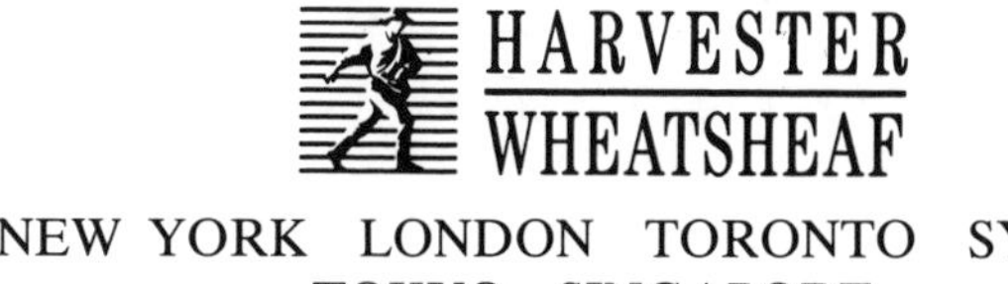

NEW YORK LONDON TORONTO SYDNEY
TOKYO SINGAPORE

First published 1993 by
Harvester Wheatsheaf
Campus 400, Maylands Avenue
Hemel Hempstead
Hertfordshire, HP2 7EZ
A division of
Simon & Schuster International Group

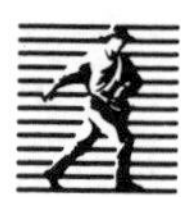

Typeset in Linotron Times 10/12pt
by Columns Design & Production Services Ltd., Reading, UK

Printed and bound in Great Britain by
Biddles Ltd, Guildford and King's Lynn

British Library Cataloguing in Publication Data

A catalogue record for this book is available from the British Library

ISBN 0–7450–1184–5 (hbk)
ISBN 0–7450–1247–7 (pbk)

1 2 3 4 5 97 96 95 94 93

For our sisters: Dais, Noreen and Valerie

Contents

Acknowledgements

We have many grateful acknowledgements to make. The idea for the book and the theoretical model it proposes were conceived by the first two authors in the mid 1980s, but responsibility for the research we report is shared with many other people. The research on pregnancy outcome was funded by grants to Lyn Quine and Derek Rutter from the Rowntree Foundation, the Department of Health, and the University of Kent at Canterbury. Funding for the research on breast cancer screening came from the South East Thames Regional Health Authority and the National Breast Screening Programme. These grants were made to Michael Calnan, Stuart Field, Derek Rutter and Michael Vaile. The research on motorcycling safety was funded by a contract to Derek Rutter and Lyn Quine from the Department of Transport. Sarah Gowen and Robert Hayward collected parts of the data on pregnancy outcome in Chapter 2. Barbara Wall and Kristin Wade were the principal research assistants on the breast screening studies reported in Chapter 3. David Chesham was research fellow on the motorcycling safety study reported in Chapter 4. We thank them all. We would also like to thank Jo Lemon for producing the entire manuscript and keeping us in order.

Permission to reproduce the following figures is gratefully acknowledged. Figure 1.1: OPCS (1990), Longitudinal Study, LS No. 5, OPCS; Figure 1.2: Brown GW and Harris T (1978), *The Social Origins of Depression: A study of psychiatric disorder in women*, Tavistock; Figure 1.3: Ley P (1988), *Communicating with Patients*, Chapman & Hall; Figure 1.4: Frederikson L (1992), PhD thesis The role of information in medical consultation, University of York; Figure 1.6: Fishbein M and Ajzen I (1975), *Belief, Attitude, Intention and Behavior*, Addison-Wesley; Figure 2.1: Macfarlane A and Mugford M (1984), *Birth Counts: Statistics of pregnancy and childbirth,* OPCS; Table 3.1: Vessey M (1991), *Breast Cancer Screening 1991: Evidence and experience since the Forrest Report*, NHSPSP Publications; Figure 3.4: Forrest P (1986), *Breast Cancer Screening*, DHSS; Figure 3.7: Ajzen I (1988), *Attitudes, Personality and Behavior*, Open University Press.

Chapter 1

Introduction

Outline, plan and a theoretical approach

Health psychology has existed as a recognizable discipline for perhaps ten years. Only very recently, however, have the implications of *social* psychology begun to be explored in the health literature, and this is one of the first books to include Social Psychology in its title. Many approaches to health are possible within the framework of social psychology, but our own focus is deliberately narrow. For us, the key issue is how social psychological variables affect outcomes, and in particular how they *mediate* between 'social inputs' and outcomes, where 'social inputs' are social class, education, age, and so on. The purpose of this book is to examine the social psychological mechanisms by which inputs are turned into outcomes, and to trace the causal pathways.

The three central chapters present our own research – on pregnancy outcome, breast cancer and motorcycling safety. The structure of the three chapters is the same. We begin by outlining the published epidemiological data to identify the scale of the problems we shall address and to draw out the principal social inputs we shall examine in our empirical research. In the case of pregnancy outcome (Chapter 2), the key outcomes we identify are infant mortality and low birthweight, pregnancy complications and satisfaction with services. In breast cancer (Chapter 3), there are well-established patterns of relationships between social inputs and mortality, incidence and survival, and among the most important are age, social class, marriage and motherhood. As to motorcycling (Chapter 4), the key outcome is accident involvement, and the leading inputs are sex, age and riding experience.

From an examination of the epidemiological data and the issues for social psychological mediation they indicate, each of the three chapters turns to a review of the existing published research on the issues. In Chapter 2, the route from social class to outcome is traced through life-events and social support, emotion and cognition, coping strategies and behaviour. In Chapter 3, attendance for regular breast screening is shown to be an important link between inputs and outcomes, and the literature highlights the part that beliefs, expectations and anxiety play in attendance. In Chapter 4, a variety of links are explored between accident involvement and age, sex and motorcycling experience, notably through the mediation of attitudes and risk perception, and appropriate and inappropriate behaviours. Each of the chapters is thus concerned to identify its own key mediators, and the particular mediators we emphasize will differ from chapter to chapter.

To return to this first chapter, the section that follows offers a definition of health and outlines some of the ways in which it can be measured. After that, we shall present a review of the social psychological literature on health. In line with our overall theoretical approach, the structure of the review will emphasize social inputs and health outcomes, and the mediators that link them, and we shall concentrate on the mediators that have received the most attention: life-events and social support, knowledge and information, emotion, cognitive dispositions, coping and appropriate and inappropriate behaviours. The final section of the chapter will draw the evidence together, and will pave the way for our own investigations in Chapters 2, 3 and 4 by combining the findings of the review into a theoretical model. Chapter 5 will bring together the results of our whole programme and will explore the implications of our approach for theory, and for policy and practice.

Health: definitions and indices

Perhaps the most difficult tasks in writing about social psychology and health are to define what we mean by health and to decide how to measure it. The World Health Organization, in its 1948 constitution, proposed that health should be seen as 'a state of complete physical, mental and social well-being, and not merely the absence of disease or infirmity'. At the heart of the definition lay the individual and positive well-being. Thirty years later, however, in launching its 'Global Strategy for Health for All by the Year 2000', WHO spoke of 'the attainment by all citizens of the world by the year 2000 of a level of health that will permit them to lead a socially and economically productive life'. Well-being had been replaced by absence from illness and infirmity, and the individual had given way to the global.

In 1978, WHO went on to urge that the way for governments to strive for the goal of health for all was through primary care. Each nation should have a stated health policy, with strategies and plans of action to launch and sustain primary health care as part of a comprehensive health system. There should be international co-operation to develop and implement health systems based on primary care throughout the world, but with particular emphasis on developing countries. There should be national, regional and global monitoring and evaluation of the strategy. Governments responded in a variety of ways, and one of the most recent statements from the UK Department of Health – a consultative document published in 1991, called *The Health of the Nation* (Department of Health, 1991) – stated as its ideal that each person should lead a 'physically and mentally healthy life well into old age'. Primary care was seen as an important means of reaching that ideal, but the difficulty was to find yardsticks by which to measure achievement.

WHO's solution was to propose twelve criteria, which together make up its 'global indicators' for monitoring and evaluating the 'Health for All' strategy.

1. Health for all has received endorsement as policy at the highest official level.
2. Mechanisms for involving people in the implementation of strategies have been formed or strengthened, and are actually functioning.
3. At least 5 per cent of the gross national product is spent on health.

4. A reasonable percentage of the national health expenditure is devoted to local health care.
5. Resources are equitably distributed.
6. The number of developing countries with well-defined strategies for health for all, accompanied by explicit resource allocations, whose needs for external resources are receiving sustained support from more affluent countries [is substantial].
7. Primary health care is available to the whole population, with at least the following: safe water in the home or within 15 minutes' walking distance, and adequate sanitary facilities in the home or immediate vicinity; immunization against diphtheria, tetanus, whooping-cough, measles, poliomyelitis and tuberculosis; local health care, including availability of at least twenty essential drugs, within one hour's walk or travel; trained personnel for attending pregnancy and childbirth, and caring for children up to at least one year of age.
8. The nutritional status of children is adequate, in that at least 90 per cent of newborn infants have a birth weight of at least 2,500 g; at least 90 per cent of children have a weight-for-age that corresponds to the standard reference values adopted by WHO.
9. The infant mortality rate for all identifiable subgroups is below 50 per 1,000 live births.
10. Life expectancy at birth is over 60 years.
11. The adult literacy rate for both men and women exceeds 70 per cent.
12. The gross national product per capita exceeds US$500.

An important feature of WHO's criteria was that several were *outcome* measures – 8, 9 and 10, for example. We too shall concentrate on outcomes as our principal index of health, and we shall be concerned with two main types. The first are 'hard' outcomes, such as mortality and morbidity, and the second are 'soft' outcomes, such as psychological adjustment to illness and satisfaction with services. We shall also be concerned with behaviours that are predicted by social inputs and social psychological mediators, and that go on to influence outcomes. Outcomes, we believe, are among the most sensitive indices of health for social psychologists to address, and they will therefore provide the focus for our empirical work. Chapter 2 will examine a 'soft' outcome, satisfaction with maternity care, the birth experience and medical communications; Chapter 3 will concentrate on a behaviour, attendance for breast cancer screening, which the evidence suggests is linked to a 'hard' outcome, reduced mortality; and Chapter 4 will examine both a 'hard' outcome, accident involvement, and a set of behaviours that lead to it, namely unsafe riding.

Inputs, mediators and outcomes: a review

Social inputs

It is well established in the epidemiological literature that health outcomes are closely related to social inputs. In Britain, one of the most useful sources of information is the Office of Population Censuses and Surveys (OPCS), which publishes annual statistics on both mortality and morbidity. Among the principal facts in the most recent statistics are these (OPCS, 1991a, 1991b). Women can expect to live longer than men. Life expectancy at birth is estimated to be 78 years for women and 73 years for men, and women who reach 80 can expect to live a further eight years on average, against six for men. There are almost 230,000 women over 90 in England and Wales, against fewer than 50,000 men. Death rates for males are higher for every age group than for females – including children – and there are marked sex and age differences in causes of death. For both men and women, diseases of the circulatory system (including heart attacks and strokes) account for almost half of all deaths, and cancer comes second. For men and women combined, heart disease is the most common cause of death in people aged 65 and over, while cancer is the most common cause for people aged 15 to 64. Morbidity, too, shows marked effects, with self-defined longstanding illness slightly more common in women than men (33 per cent against 31 per cent). People who are widowed, separated or divorced are much more likely to report longstanding illness than are those who are single or married. Women visit their GP six times a year on average, against four times for men, and 12 per cent go into hospital as an in-patient at some time in a given year, against 8 per cent of men.

Of all the social inputs, the one that has received the most attention in the literature is social class. In Britain, the most common way of classifying people is by occupation, using what is now called the *Standard Occupational Classification* (OPCS, 1990). There are six groups: professional (I); employers and managers (II); intermediate and junior non-manual (IIInm); skilled manual (IIIm); semi-skilled manual and personal services (IV); and unskilled manual (V). Married women are classified according to their husband's occupation. The outcome measure examined most frequently has been mortality, and much the most influential contribution to the literature has been the seminal 'Black Report', published in 1980 (Black, 1980).

The Black Report (1980)

Black's data for mortality came from OPCS, and were based on the Occupational Mortality Decennial Supplement for 1970–2 (OPCS, 1978). When the number of deaths in each social class was divided by the number of people in the class, the rates showed a steadily increasing gradient from Class I to Class V. For men the rates were 3.98 in Class I to 9.88 in Class V, and for women they were 2.15 to 5.31. In other words, the number of people who died at the bottom of the social scale was 2½ times the number who 'ought' to have died, given the number of people in each class and the number who died at the top.

Ten years on, the divide was wider still. Again using the OPCS Decennial Supplement, Marmot and McDowall (1986) examined particular *causes* of death, and compared 1970–2 with 1979–83. Occupational groups were collapsed into two bands, middle class (I–IIInm) and working class (IIIm–V), and standardized mortality ratios for the two bands were compared for the two periods. For men, for all causes of death combined, the ratio for middle class to working class was 0.77 in 1970–2 and 0.69 in 1979–83. For the separate causes of death the authors examined, the figures were 0.58 and 0.50 for lung cancer, 0.90 and 0.76 for coronary heart disease, and 0.80 and 0.63 for strokes. The analysis for women produced similar results, and the conclusion was the same: in ten years the social divide had widened. Detailed accounts of the changes are to be found in Macintyre (1986), Wilkinson (1986), Whitehead (1987), Goldblatt (1989, 1990), Smith, Bartley and Blane (1990) and Blane, Smith and Bartley (1990).

Theoretical accounts of social inequalities

If Black's first achievement was to bring together the evidence of inequalities into a coherent body of knowledge, his second was to outline the possible interpretations and to debate their very different implications. There were three main theories in the literature. The first was that the reported inequalities were artefacts of the ways in which social class, and perhaps inequalities too, were defined and measured (LeGrand, 1985; Illsley, 1986). Changes over time in the comparison of occupational groupings, in the criteria for assigning people to categories and in the personnel making the assignments could all lead to apparent inequalities if people who were unhealthy at Time 2 were placed in a lower category than at Time 1. The second theory was that inequalities were real rather than apparent, and occurred because people who were unhealthy or potentially unhealthy were 'selected' for low-status occupations or 'drifted downwards' into them, while healthy people were selected or climbed upwards (Illsley, 1980, 1986; Stern, 1983; LeGrand, 1986; Illsley and LeGrand, 1987). The third theory was that people at the bottom of the social scale suffered material deprivation, which affected their health behaviours and outcomes. The 'strongest' form of the theory was structural and said that material deprivation affected outcomes *directly*. For example, people at the bottom of the scale worked in occupations with high levels of industrial accidents, and lived in overcrowded housing which might be damp, and the individual played little if any part in mediating the effects. The second version of the theory said that material deprivation operated *indirectly*, and had its effects through the individual's behaviour. For example, lack of money prevented people taking up services because time and travel were expensive, and similar arguments applied to diet, healthy leisure, and so on. The third form of the theory was that material deprivation itself *produced* inappropriate behaviours, which in turn were responsible for the observed negative outcomes.

Black concluded that 'it is in some form or forms of the "materialist" approach that the best answer lies' (Black, 1980, p. 120), and it is probably fair to say that the majority of writers agree (see, for example, the reviews by Macintyre, 1986, 1988; Wilkinson, 1986; the British Medical Association, 1987; Hart, 1987; the Health Promotion and Research Trust, 1987; Whitehead, 1987). Nevertheless, the artefactual and selection theories have been very difficult to dismiss satisfactorily in the case of adult mortality – though not infant mortality, as we shall see in Chapter 2 – for proper tests need prospective longitudinal data and none has existed. Now, however, the position has changed, for a number of longitudinal studies have begun to report their findings.

Prospective longitudinal research

Three studies in particular deserve attention, and all of them are from Britain. The first is the OPCS Longitudinal Study. From the 1971 Census, a random sample of the population of England and Wales was taken, 1 per cent of all males and 1 per cent of all females, and the resulting 500,000 are being monitored from official records until they die, so that significant demographic and health changes can be charted (Figure 1.1). One of the purposes of the study is to examine mortality by social class, using the person's recorded occupation in the original 1971 Census, so that the artefactual problems identified by Black can be overcome. Since the census is repeated every ten years, it will also be possible to test social selection theories as the person's occupational status and health status change. Already, the first waves of data support the pattern demonstrated by the Decennial Supplements: inequalities exist and are widening. For example, a comparison of men from Class V in 1971 with men from Class I, using standardized mortality ratios, shows differences of 1.41 : 1 in 1971–5, 1.86 : 1 in 1976–81, and 1.79 : 1 in 1982–5 (Goldblatt, 1989). The differences are smaller than in the Decennial Supplements, but the pattern is the same. It is safe to conclude that artefact was not a sufficient explanation for Black's original findings.

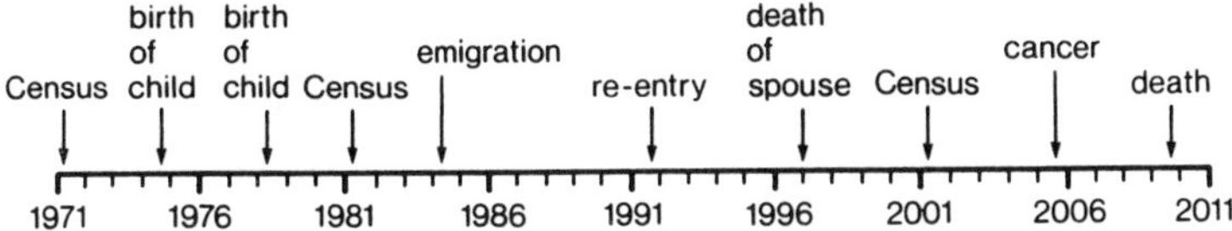

Figure 1.1 Examples of the spacing of LS records in time

The second study is the British Regional Heart Study. In 1979–80 a random sample of 7,735 British men aged 40–59 was selected from general practices, and all were sent an invitation to take part in the study. A total of 78 per cent accepted, and each volunteer completed a physical examination and a health screening questionnaire, which included a measure of social class. The men have since been monitored continually for evidence of heart disease, and significant effects were found even after the first six years of follow-up (Pocock *et al.*, 1987). More than 300 men had suffered a heart attack (not always fatal) at some time during the six years, and the ratio for working-class men to middle-class men was 1.44 : 1. Part of the difference was attributable to *pre-existing* differences between the two groups in known risk factors – age, smoking, blood pressure and blood cholesterol – but there was still a ratio of 1.24 : 1 when the differences were controlled statistically. It remains to be seen whether the divide will widen as the period of follow-up lengthens, but already it is substantial.

The third study has become known as the Whitehall Study of civil servants. The findings we have examined so far have come from coarse-grained comparisons between the top of the social scale and the bottom. The purpose of the Whitehall Study was to take a group of people who were all in one occupation in one geographical location and examine whether even *within* so narrow a (predominantly middle-class) band there was still a gradient to be found. In 1967–9, 17,530 civil servants working in Whitehall were identified, and their grade was noted – from 'administrative' at the top, to 'professional and executive', 'clerical' and 'other' (mainly messengers and unskilled manual workers). Measures were taken at the outset of a variety of physical, medical and behavioural indices, and the men were then monitored over time. In the first ten-year follow-up, the familiar gradient was found once again, with mortality rates more than three times higher at the bottom than at the top. The age-adjusted ratio was greatest for lung cancer (7.2 : 1) but was present for all the major causes of death, including coronary heart disease (2.8 : 1), which accounted for the greatest number of deaths in all, over 40 per cent (Marmot, Shipley and Rose, 1984; Marmot, 1986).

The Whitehall Study is very important. In common with both the previous prospective longitudinal studies we have discussed, it eliminates artefactual bias, yet finds significant inequalities. Indeed, despite so narrow a sample and the shared location, some of the ratios are the greatest we have encountered. The implication is that health inequalities have both specific and non-specific causes. A familiar example of specific causes, those that predispose to *particular* illnesses and causes of death, is smoking. In the Whitehall Study, as elsewhere, smoking was much higher at the bottom of the scale than at the top and it no doubt contributed significantly to the marked difference in deaths from lung cancer. However, coronary heart disease, for which smoking is again an established risk factor, showed a steep gradient even among *non*-smokers, as we have seen. Indeed, a ratio of over 2 : 1 between the bottom and the top remained when *every* risk factor that had been measured was removed statistically. In other words, the pattern must have been caused in part by *non-specific* factors, those that produce susceptibility to illness in general and not just to individual illnesses in particular.

The important task now is to identify what the factors may be. According to Marmot, they will prove to be both biological and social. One possibility, for example, is height, which is an index of both genetic and early environmental influences, and is known to predispose (inversely) to morbidity and mortality in general. The Whitehall Study found that mortality in the shortest men was 1.36 times greater than in the tallest – and, just as the argument requires, men at the top of the civil service grades were on average taller than those at the bottom. Whatever the eventual explanation of social class differences in health, it must, Marmot concludes, incorporate 'not only biological understanding but also an insight into the social causes of differences in environment and personal behaviour which have so great an effect on health and mortality' (Marmot, Shipley and Rose, 1984, p. 1006).

Stressful life-events

From social inputs we turn now to mediators, variables through which we believe inputs have their effects upon outcomes. The first we consider are stressful life-events. Interest in the area began with the work of Hinkle and Wolff (1957), who concluded from longitudinal studies that 'clusters of illness most often appear when a person is having difficulty adapting to his environment as perceived by him'. They suggested that inherent differences in adaptive capacities, and different levels of difficulty encountered, determined the amount of illness individuals experienced. Both physical and mental illness were implicated.

Systematic study of the role of stressful events in the onset of illness was made possible by the development of a method for assessing life-events. This was the Social Readjustment Rating Scale (Holmes and Rahe, 1967). Holmes and Rahe argued that the important attribute of life-events was *the amount of adaptation or readjustment* they required the individual to make to his or her lifestyle, rather than the psychological meaning of the event. Although it has subsequently been modified by others (Dohrenwend *et al.*, 1978), the original hypothesis generated an extensive body of research. Findings from numerous studies found a modest but significant relationship between major life-events and the onset and occurrence of many medical and psychological disorders (Rabkin and Streuning, 1976; Dohrenwend and Dohrenwend, 1978).

Methods of measurement

There have been two main strategies for eliciting the life-events of subjects. The first, as we have noted, originated with the Social Readjustment Rating Scale of Holmes and Rahe. The respondent is presented with an inventory of events, and endorses those items that describe his experiences in the specified period (typically the previous twelve months). The procedure takes 15–20 minutes. Each item carries a particular weight or score (previously obtained by reference to a separate sample) and these are summed to give an individual's total score. What is regarded as an event is thus determined beforehand, and the assumption is made that a given experience has the same impact on all individuals, irrespective of circumstance and personality. The original list has been used and modified by many researchers (Paykel, Prusoff and Uhlenhuth, 1971; Henderson, Byrne and Duncan-Jones, 1981).

The second approach to measurement was developed by Brown and Harris (1978) and involves the use of a semi-structured interview with questions designed to elicit possible events in different domains of the subject's life. The interview may take 2–3 hours. When the history has been collected, the interviewer presents vignettes of the events to a panel of raters. In order to avoid contamination of variables, raters are given only limited information about the subject's social background and none at all about his or her psychiatric state or actual response to the events. They then decide upon the severity of each event and the impact it is likely to have had on the individual. The rationale behind the procedure is explained by Brown (1974), and Shrout (1981) provides a useful critique of the theory and assumptions underlying the method. The approach assumes that it is the distressing quality of the event and its long-term threat that is important, rather than the adaptation required, and that a given event may not cause the same level of distress to each person. This variability of impact had been seen to be a major problem with the Social Readjustment Rating Scale.

Methodological difficulties in researching life-events

Early investigators had hoped that life-events would explain much of the aetiology of illness, particularly psychiatric disorders. However, as Tennant and Andrews (1978) have observed, these initial hopes have somewhat faded because of the considerable difficulties in measuring exposure to stressful experiences and assessing their effects. A preoccupation with method has emerged, and reviews by Sarason and Spielberger (1979),

Dohrenwend and Dohrenwend (1981) and Paykel (1983) provide accounts of the difficulties. They include problems with the characteristics of the measures themselves, such as representativeness of items, item weighting schemes and their psychometric properties (Rabkin and Streuning, 1976; Cleary, 1980; Lei and Skinner, 1980); problems concerning the possible existence of moderating variables in the stress–disorder relationship, such as personality variables, coping strategies and social support (Dohrenwend and Dohrenwend, 1978; Cleary, 1980; Henderson, 1980); problems of ensuring that reports of life-events are not contaminated by the individual's emotional state; and problems of demonstrating causality, which requires precise dating of the life-event in relation to the onset of illness (Henderson *et al.*, 1981; Creed, 1985). In addition, recent investigations have proposed that relatively minor difficulties – daily hassles – may also play a part in the stress–illness equation (Kanner *et al.*, 1981; Lazarus, 1984).

Many studies have shown an association between life-events and illness using *cross-sectional* data (Dohrenwend and Dohrenwend, 1978; Creed, 1985). However, these do little to advance understanding about *causal* relationships since they simply confirm that people with symptoms report more life-events than do healthy people. In order to infer causality it is necessary to use a *prospective* longitudinal design in which exposure to adversity is measured before the onset of symptoms – though even then the positive association may be due to personality traits, which may predispose an individual both to severe life-events and to illness. Even in prospective studies, life-events typically explain only 10 per cent or so of the variance in morbidity (Rabkin and Streuning, 1976), which means that 90 per cent of the variance is not accounted for. An alternative way of expressing the contribution is the relative risk statistic, which is the ratio of the incidence of a particular illness in those exposed and those not exposed to life-events (Paykel, 1978). Brown *et al.* (1986b), for example, reported a relative risk of 14 for depression in women exposed to a provoking factor, that is, they were 14 times more likely to become depressed than women not exposed to a provoking factor. For statistical reasons, however, even relative risks that high are compatible with as little as 10 per cent of variance being explained.

The evidence

What evidence is there that stressful life-events play a causal role in physical and psychiatric illness? The evidence from prospective studies is more valid and reliable than that of cross-sectional studies, as we have suggested already, since prospective designs do much to eliminate the possibility of spuriously positive associations, and thus provide potentially more powerful evidence for a *causal* association. The evidence from prospective studies so far is mixed.

Psychiatric illness. The majority of the literature has investigated *psychiatric* illness, and the disorders that have received the most attention are neurosis and depression. Tennant (1983) reviewed ten prospective studies and found that only two revealed positive findings, those by Theorell, Lind and Floderus (1975) and Henderson *et al.* (1981). The implication was that life-events do not have any substantial causal role in either neurotic or depressive illness, but Tennant advocated more emphasis on prospective designs, more sensitive measures of stress with short follow-up periods and the inclusion of personality measures – which in Henderson's study had been much the most important source of variance. Finlay-Jones (1988) in a later review, on the other hand, concluded that life-events involving *a loss* are an important cause of depressive illness and its outcome, and also of suicidal behaviour and mania. There was evidence too that life-events involving danger contributed to the onset of anxiety states. The literature on depression was also reviewed by Bebbington (1985), who concluded that the evidence may be stronger for mild states of depression than for more severe states, and that when events do lead to depression they take place only two or three months before the onset of symptoms.

One of the difficulties for life-events researchers has been that life-events do not always lead to illness. The work of Brown and his colleagues has been influential in demonstrating that other variables, particularly vulnerability factors, interact with adversity. Brown argues that certain provoking agents determine when an episode of depression takes place, and the most significant are severe life-events, usually involving an important loss or disappointment. A second provoking agent that plays a less important role is on-going major difficulties. Brown estimates that about 60 per cent of episodes of depression among psychiatric patients and 80–90 per cent among women in the general population are brought about by stressful life-events. However, their effects are greatly influenced by the presence of vulnerability factors, which increase risk in the presence of a provoking agent and have little or no effect without them. There are three major vulnerability factors, Brown argues: lack of an intimate tie with a husband, having three or more children under the age of 14 living at home, and loss of a mother before the age of 11. Lack of employment may also act as a vulnerability factor under certain circumstances (Brown and Harris, 1978; Brown, 1987). Another set of factors, symptom formation factors, influence only the form and severity of the depression. Brown's model is presented in Figure 1.2 (Brown and Harris, 1978, p. 48).

The other disorder to have received attention is schizophrenia, and again the evidence is mixed. In a detailed review, Tennant (1985) concluded that life-events may precipitate hospital admission of schizophrenic patients, that events may be associated with affective or neurotic symptoms in schizophrenia, and that there may be an association between life-events and expressed emotion, leading to relapse. However, he found the evidence that life-events play a causal role in the *onset* of schizophrenia was less conclusive, with only one methodologically sound study,

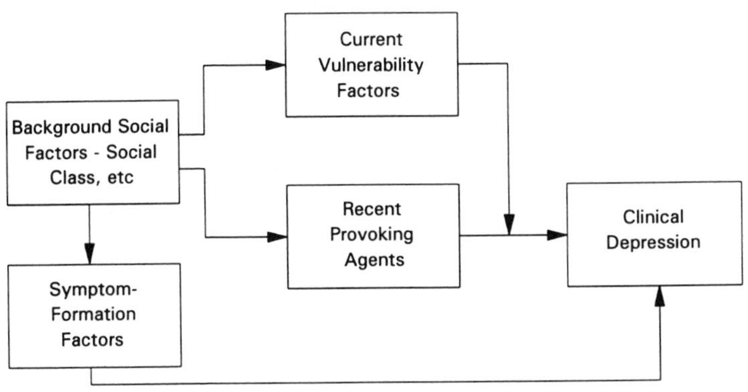

Figure 1.2 Social origins of depression: Brown and Harris (1978)

by Brown and Birley (1968), finding an effect. In contrast, recent cross-cultural research carried out by investigators in seven countries under the auspices of the World Health Organization (Day *et al.*, 1987) found that life-events do contribute to the onset of acute episodes of schizophrenia and cluster in the two or three weeks prior to onset of illness. The issues remain to be resolved.

Physical illness. The onset of physical illness has frequently been shown to be preceded by a significant increase in stress (as measured by the use of life-event scales). In cross-sectional studies, the relationship has been documented for general ill health by numerous researchers, including Rahe, McKean and Arthur (1967), Cline and Chosey (1972) and Holmes and Masuda (1974), though at least two prospective studies have *failed* to find an effect (Theorell *et al.*, 1975; Goldberg and Comstock, 1976). The evidence for specific illness is less satisfactory, but a relationship has been claimed in myocardial infarction (Theorell and Rahe, 1971; Connolly, 1976), tuberculosis (Holmes *et al.*, 1957), acute glaucoma (Cohen and Hajioff, 1972), inguinal hernia (Rahe *et al.*, 1964), rheumatoid arthritis (Heisel, 1972), subarachnoid haemorrhage (Penrose, 1972); appendicitis (Creed, 1981); the common cold (Tolman *et al.*, 1980); and leukaemia (Rabkin and Streuning, 1976). It is well established that increased illness follows bereavement and natural disaster (Parkes, 1970). Life-events researchers claim that stressors are cumulative, and that the impact of less serious events such as moving house or changes of occupation when taken together may be as pathogenic as bereavement (Holmes and Masuda, 1974). The evidence has been reviewed by Creed (1985).

Social support

The notion that social support might contribute to mental and physical health has its origins in a series of theories about social networks (Litwak and Szelenyi, 1969), social disorganization (Leighton *et al.*, 1963), and the basic human need for social transactions (Maslow, 1968). In the mid-1970s three major papers were published which reviewed the mounting evidence (Cassel,

1976; Cobb, 1976; Kaplan, Cassel and Gore, 1977). The protective effects of social support were reported for numerous disease outcomes, including overall mortality, pregnancy outcome, psychiatric illness, suicide, accidents, recovery from illness and death from chronic disease (Broadhead *et al.*, 1983). Since these papers there has been a huge body of research on the relationship of social support to both physical and psychiatric morbidity (for reviews see Mueller, 1980; Greenblatt, Becerra and Serafetinides, 1982; Thoits, 1982; Broadhead *et al.*, 1983; Monroe, 1983; Schradle and Dougher, 1985; Alloway and Bebbington, 1987). Several hypotheses have emerged. The original hypothesis was that social support provided a buffering effect against adversity but had no independent effect in the absence of adversity (Dean and Lin, 1977). However, research by Henderson *et al.* (1978a, 1978b) suggested that it might have a direct and independent effect on mental and/or physical health regardless of whether adversity was experienced. A third version of the theory suggested that social support has a therapeutic effect after the onset of a particular disorder, shortening the episode and reducing symptoms. Lastly, it has been suggested that social support could be deleterious for some members of the community, particularly elderly people (Lowenthal, 1964).

Definitions of social support

Although the construct of social support has been a central variable in stress–illness research, there has been considerable disagreement about its definition or functions. Cassel (1976) defines social support in terms of the simple presence of others, while Nuckolls, Cassel and Kaplan (1972) see it in terms of the availability of 'psycho-social assets'. Cobb's influential conceptualization considers social support as 'information leading the subject to believe that (1) he is cared for and loved; (2) esteemed and valued; and (3) belongs to a network of communication and mutual obligation' (Cobb, 1976).

More recent attempts at analyzing the functions of social support argue for a refinement of current conceptualizations and measurements in ways that refer to the nature and type of support, the sources of support, and both the availability and adequacy of the relationships. Thoits (1982) has recommended a definition based on Kaplan *et al.* (1977): 'the degree to which an individual's basic needs for affection, approval, belonging and security are gratified through interaction with others.' These needs, according to Kaplan, may be met by the provision of socio-emotional aid (affection, sympathy, understanding, acceptance and esteem from significant others) or by the provision of instrumental aid (advice and information, help with family responsibilities, financial help). These are similar to the six functions of social relationships identified by Weiss (1974), which are attachment, social integration, an opportunity for nurturing others, reassurance of personal worth, a sense of reliable alliance and guidance from others. A further typology, which has the attraction of being a mnemonic, is that of Kahn and Antonucci (1980): affect (someone expressing affection); affirmation (someone saying they are of like mind); and aid (help and advice). A similar construct is Hinde's triad of affect, cognition and behaviour (Hinde, 1979).

A number of writers have considered the mechanisms by which social support may influence health both directly and by buffering. Integration into a social network may mean that individuals experience greater attachment and higher self-esteem, and have a feeling of greater personal control. Each of these factors might be protective through a variety of physiological mechanisms, for example by working on the immune system (O'Leary, 1990; Kaplan, 1991), or by making changes to lifestyle. Social support may also have direct effects by providing an individual with a valued social role, a positive social identity, or experiences of mastery and self-efficacy (Thoits, 1985). In contrast, it may serve to buffer the effects of severe life stressors by redirecting the stressor or by regulating the emotional distress caused by it (Gore, 1981; Cohen and McKay, 1984).

The measurement of social support

The measurement of social support has posed a considerable challenge. There have been four main approaches. First, sociodemographic variables such as marital status have been used as indicators of social relationships (Lynch, 1977). Second, indices of social support have been derived from a small number of questionnaire items about marital status, living arrangements, contact with others at home and at work, and involvement in community activities (Berkman and Syme, 1979). Third, measures of specific aspects of social relationships have been used (Brown, Bhrolcháin and Harris, 1975; Brown and Harris, 1978). Brown and his colleagues, for example, have produced a Self Evaluation and Social Support interview to investigate the existence of close, confiding relationships (Brown *et al.*, 1986a). A fourth method has been to construct purpose-built instruments for measuring the availability and adequacy of social relationships and what they provide for the subject. Reviews of the various measures have been published by Orth-Gomér and Undén (1987) and O'Reilly (1988).

From the four main approaches to measurement, a number of published scales have emerged. The most frequently used are the Social Support Questionnaire (Schaefer, Coyne and Lazarus, 1981), the Social Relationship and Activity Scale (House, 1981), the Interview Schedule for Social Interaction (Henderson *et al.*, 1980), and the Short Social Support Scale (Funch, Marshall and Gebhardt, 1986). Satisfactory reliability has been established for each of the instruments, though problems of validation have arisen (Henderson, Byrne and Duncan-Jones 1981). For example, it is difficult to determine whether the measures provide a true reflection of the individual's support or whether they are confounded by personality factors and mood states – which may influence a person's ability to establish and maintain relationships and also the way he describes and evaluates his support. A further problem is that social support can be confounded by recent life-events, for people who have suffered severe life-events will thereby often have suffered recent losses of social support. Ways must be found to disentangle the effects, though a number of writers have acknowledged that to measure the components of social support in a way that keeps them free of personality and other attributes may be logically impossible. They advocate that a better approach is to mount intervention studies, in which the variables of interest are manipulated systematically (Henderson, 1984).

The evidence

The evidence for a relationship between social support and *physical* health has been reviewed by Berkman (1984, 1986). Berkman argues that there is increasing evidence from prospective epidemiological investigations that social support reduces mortality. The relationship is stronger for men than women, but the mechanisms by which social support has its effects are poorly understood. Berkman suggests that a shorter life and poor social relationships may both be related to personality traits, of which neuroticism and anxiety are among the most important.

In *mental* health, there is again relatively little prospective data, but a plethora of cross-sectional studies has been published showing a relationship with social support (Cohen and Sokolovsky, 1978; Henderson *et al.*, 1978a, 1978b). However, the evidence is open to a number of interpretations, as we have already hinted. One possibility is that poor social support causes mental ill-health, while another is that people who are depressed withdraw socially, or simply have a gloomy view of their social networks. Of the prospective studies, some have tested for a buffering effect and some for an independent effect, and equivocal findings have emerged (Henderson *et al.*, 1981; Pearlin *et al.*, 1981; Lin and Dean, 1984; Brown *et al.*, 1986a, 1986b). Henderson's study found an association between reported inadequacy of social support and the onset of symptoms of neurotic illness in the presence of life-events. However, a measure of neuroticism in the same study accounted for much more of the variance in subsequent symptoms (69 per cent). Brown's ambitious study, on the other hand, based on a sample of 395 working-class women, found that for married women the existence of a confiding relationship measured at Time 1 was not associated with a lower risk of depression in the succeeding year. In contrast, single mothers were less likely to become depressed if they had access to socially supportive relationships. To try to resolve the differences between the two approaches, Henderson and Brown subsequently worked together, and produced a critical review (Henderson and Brown, 1988). The main emphasis of the paper was methodological.

As we saw earlier, Henderson has argued that the best way to disentangle cause and effect is to mount intervention studies in which social support is manipulated systematically. Impressive evidence has come recently from intervention studies in pregnancy (Klaus *et al.*, 1986; Flint and Poulengeris, 1987; Oakley, 1988; Elbourne and Oakley, 1990). In the most recent of the studies, by Oakley, Rajan and Grant (1990), 509 women with a history of low birthweight took part. Half received extra social support in addition to standard antenatal care, and half did not. The extra support was given by four research midwives, who offered 24-hour telephone contact and a programme of home visits. Babies in the intervention group had a mean birthweight 38 g higher than the babies in the control group, and there were fewer very low-birthweight babies. More women in the control group were admitted to hospital during pregnancy, while spontaneous onset of labour and spontaneous vaginal delivery were more common in the intervention group, who also required less epidural anaesthesia. Babies in the intervention group required less intensive care and special neonatal care, and were significantly healthier in the early weeks, as were their mothers. There could be little doubt that the effects had been caused by the manipulation, and social support was thus shown to be a powerful variable.

Emotional factors

One of the more consistent findings in the literature on mental health has been that people with emotional disorders, such as depression and anxiety, have an elevated risk of mortality (Tsuang and Simpson, 1985; Lieberman and Coburn, 1986; Zilber, Schufman and Lerner, 1989). Most of the evidence comes from patients in treatment or from highly selected non-patient groups, usually male industrial workers, and there is remarkable consistency across studies and across time. There is also evidence from community-based epidemiological investigations. Here, subjects are selected on the basis of their prior mental and physical illness and other characteristics, and therefore constitute a more representative sample both of the communities in which they live and of the full spectrum of illnesses. The findings this time have been more equivocal.

Depression

From treatment and non-patient studies, a clear association has been found between psychological illness and elevated risk of death. The effect is largely attributable to deaths from unnatural causes, particularly suicide (Guze and Robins, 1970), though studies in Israel and France have reported increased risk of *all-cause* mortality (Casadebaig and Quemada, 1989; Zilber *et al.*, 1989). The increased risk of suicide is in general greater for people suffering from mood or affective disorders (Black, Warrack and Winokur, 1985). Community-based studies, however, have often failed to find any relationship between psychological disorder and all-cause mortality. A wide range of locations has been sampled: Midtown Manhattan (Singer *et al.*, 1976); Missouri and Maryland (Goldberg, Comstock and Hornstra, 1979); New Haven, Connecticut (Weissman *et al.*, 1986); Piedmont, North Carolina (Fredman *et al.*, 1989); Denmark (Nielsen, Homma and Biorn-Henriksen, 1977); Alemada County, California (Roberts, Kaplan and Camacho, 1990); and Lundby, Sweden (Rorsman, Hagnell and Lanke, 1982a, 1982b). Four studies, however, *have* found an association: Stirling County, Canada (Murphy *et al.*, 1987, 1989); New Haven ECA (Bruce and Leaf, 1989); Alachua County, Florida (Markush, 1977); and Evans County, Georgia (Somervell *et al.*, 1989). In addition, two of the studies – Midtown Manhattan and Lundby, Sweden – reported an elevated risk for specific causes of death such as suicide and accidents among those depressed at baseline, but not for overall mortality.

Despite the impressive volume of the research, many of the studies, unfortunately, have suffered from small sample sizes – yielding small numbers of deaths, particularly from unnatural causes, and a lack of data on duration and severity of psychological disorder – and also from a failure to examine the known interactions of socio-economic status, somatic illness and psychological dysfunction. They also varied considerably in terms of how cases were ascertained and established. In only six of the studies were more serious forms of mental illness distinguished from milder forms. In addition, several of the studies experienced substantial attrition, the effect of which is to reduce the sample size still further, thus reducing the number of deaths available for the study. For example, in the first New Haven study, data were available at all three time-periods for only 55 per cent of the sample. Attrition may also introduce bias in the sample. Roberts *et al.* (1990) provide a critical review.

Anxiety

The evidence for an association between emotion and outcome is stronger for anxiety than for depression. There have been a number of studies that show that *patients* with anxiety suffer excess mortality and morbidity (Keehn, Goldberg and Beebe, 1974; Coryell, Noyes and Clancy, 1982; Coryell, Noyes and House, 1986; Coryell, 1988; Allgulander and Lavori, 1991). Many of the studies show also that excess mortality is largely attributable to death from unnatural causes and cardiovascular disease. Mortality from coronary heart disease, for example, is known to be especially high in people with psychiatric illness, particularly anxiety and panic disorders (see the review by Tennant, 1987).

Further evidence comes from longitudinal epidemiological studies of the general population, in Stirling County, Canada (Murphy *et al.*, 1989; Murphy, 1990) and Alachua County, Florida (Markush, 1977). The Stirling County Study, which followed up 1,003 adults for eighteen years, found that anxiety and depression both carried an increased risk of mortality, with depression having a significantly worse prognosis. When morbidity and mortality data were combined, 82 per cent of those who were depressed at the beginning of the study had a poor outcome, suggesting that depressions found in the community, where most of them remain untreated, are similar in seriousness to those seen in hospitals and out-patient clinics.

Knowledge, information and communication

Many patients complain that they are dissatisfied with the way their doctors communicate with them, and there is greater dissatisfaction with communication than with any other aspect of medical care (Cartwright, 1967; Kincey, Bradshaw and Ley, 1975; Cartwright and Anderson, 1981). The pattern is the same wherever the patient is seen – in hospital, at an out-patients department or in a community general practice – and whatever the presenting disorder (Ley, 1977, 1988). Patients complain that they are not told enough, that what they *are* told is difficult to understand and remember, and that the way they are told, the manner and emotional tone of the doctor, is unsatisfactory too. Dissatisfaction is known to be associated with patients' failing to follow the advice and treatment they are offered (Ley, 1988), and it is important to discover what causes it and what might be done to reduce it.

Affective models

Theoretical accounts in social psychology have concentrated on the doctor–patient consultation itself, and there have been two main approaches. The first has emphasized affective aspects of the interaction and is exemplified by the work of Korsch (Korsch, Gozzi and Francis, 1968; Korsch and Negrete, 1972; Korsch, 1989). Korsch was based at a children's hospital in Los Angeles, and her data came from over 800 interviews with mothers who had taken their children to a paediatric 'walk-in' clinic for acutely ill patients. Two main findings emerged. First, satisfaction with the consultation was related to the way the doctor was perceived: those who behaved in a 'friendly' way and 'understood the mother's concern' and showed 'positive' communication skills produced significantly greater satisfaction than those who did not. Second, an important part was played by the mother's expectations. Mothers who expected that the doctor would prescribe a course of treatment, for example, or would offer a diagnosis or at least examine the child, were much more satisfied when those expectations were met than when they were not. Satisfaction was thus in part a product of what the mothers brought to the encounter and not just what happened during the interaction. Similar findings emerged later from the work of Linder-Pelz (1982).

Cognitive models

The second of the theoretical approaches has emphasized cognition, and the most important contribution has come from Ley and his colleagues (Ley and Spelman, 1967; Ley, 1977, 1988). Ley argues that satisfaction with medical communications is a product of how much the patient understands of what the doctor says and how much is remembered. Satisfaction in turn leads to compliance with advice and treatment (Figure 1.3). Many experimental tests of the model have been published, and there are two main traditions, the first of which is descriptive. In

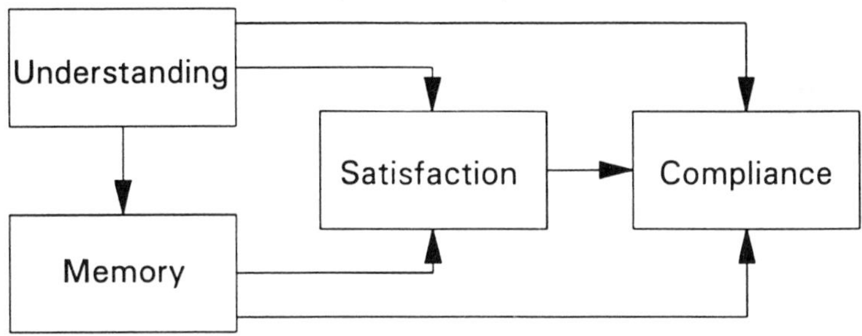

Figure 1.3 A model of satisfaction and compliance: Ley (1988)

the main, descriptive studies have used simple correlational techniques and have examined relationships between pairs of variables in the model: understanding and memory, understanding and satisfaction, memory and satisfaction, understanding and compliance, memory and compliance, and satisfaction and compliance. The strongest associations have generally been found for understanding with satisfaction, but most of the work, it should be noted, has been based on whether patients *believe* that they have understood, and not on *objective tests*. When objective tests *have* been used, notably for compliance, the correlations have generally been rather smaller (Ley, 1988).

As to *why* patients might fail to understand, two main approaches have been explored. The first is that they lack medical knowledge. In one classic study, for instance, Boyle (1970) gave multiple-choice questionnaires to people sitting in out-patient waiting rooms. Some of the questions asked them to locate a variety of vital organs, and others asked for definitions of simple medical terms. To take just a few examples, 80 per cent failed to locate the stomach properly, 60 per cent the heart and 50 per cent the kidneys, while 25 per cent defined jaundice incorrectly, 40 per cent constipation and almost 50 per cent palpitations. Similar findings have been reported more recently by Cole (1979), Segall and Roberts (1980) and Hadlow and Pitts (1991), and the implication is that a failure to understand is all that can be expected if ignorance is so widespread.

The second possible reason for poor understanding is that medical communications contain too much jargon and complexity. One popular approach has been to apply measures of reading ease, notably the Flesch formula (Flesch, 1948), to information leaflets published routinely by hospitals for patients. The Flesch formula takes into account average length of words and sentences, and a wide range of leaflets has been examined on such things as investigation procedures, a variety of illnesses and disorders, and aspects of health education. In some cases it has been estimated that almost the entire population would have difficulty understanding the information (for example, Doak and Doak, 1980), but on average the figure is around 30 per cent (Ley, 1988).

From the descriptive studies of cognitive aspects of doctor–patient communication, a number of implications have emerged for intervention, and intervention studies make up the second tradition of research. Suppose that doctors tried to correct misunderstandings and to make what they said easier to understand, and suppose that they used techniques to help their patients remember what they were told, such as structuring the information and putting the important points at the beginning or the end. Would satisfaction increase and in turn compliance? A number of programmes for training medical practitioners in communication skills have existed for some time (for example Rutter and Maguire, 1976; Pendleton and Hasler, 1983; Maguire and Faulkner, 1988a, 1988b), but the most direct evidence comes from experimental intervention studies with patients. Ley *et al.* (1976), for example, in a study of medical in-patients, found that a weekly 5-minute visit from a doctor to clarify any misunderstandings led more frequently to satisfaction with communications than either a 'placebo' visit to chat about non-medical matters or no visit at all. Many other studies have been reviewed by Ley (1988), and there is similar evidence that compliance and adherence can also be increased by improved communication (see the meta-analyses by Mazzuca, 1982; and Mullen, Green and Persinger, 1985). Indeed, it has even been found that the length of stay in hospital can be reduced (see the reviews by Anderson and Masur, 1983; and Mathews and Ridgeway, 1984). Patients in these latter studies were typically told rather more than usual about what would happen to them during an operation, for example, and they were sometimes encouraged to spend time imagining how they would feel afterwards. Speed and quality of recovery were both reported to be greater than when no special intervention was made (see the review by Devine and Cook, 1982).

Theoretical integration: input, process and outcome

From what has become an immense and detailed area of empirical research – ranging from patients' knowledge, to the quality of information doctors communicate to them, to patient satisfaction and compliance – there remains one overriding issue to confront and that is how to integrate the literature theoretically. The focus of most of the work we have reviewed has been the process of doctor–patient interaction, whether viewed from an affective or a cognitive perspective. Little attempt has been made to explore the two approaches together, or to examine the effects upon communication processes of what we have earlier called social inputs. There is, however, one major attempt at integration in the literature, and that is the work of Frederikson (1992). For Frederikson – as for Pendleton (1983) in an earlier approach – there are three levels of analysis (Figure 1.4): input (the patient's and doctor's frames of reference, expectations and knowledge); process (what happens during the consultation, particularly the exchange of information); and outcome (perceptions, diagnosis, compliance and satisfaction). For example, the patient's and doctor's frames of reference will affect the way in which they exchange information in the consultation; information exchange will in turn influence perceptions and understanding; and perceptions and understanding will lead on to satisfaction. Input, process and outcome in Frederikson's terms correspond closely to our own social inputs, mediators and outcome, and we see the model as a welcome attempt at integration, of value both for theory and for policy and practice.

Cognitive dispositions: personal control

One of the main concerns of social psychology is to try to understand how people make sense of their everyday worlds – the causes of their own and others' behaviour, and the reasons

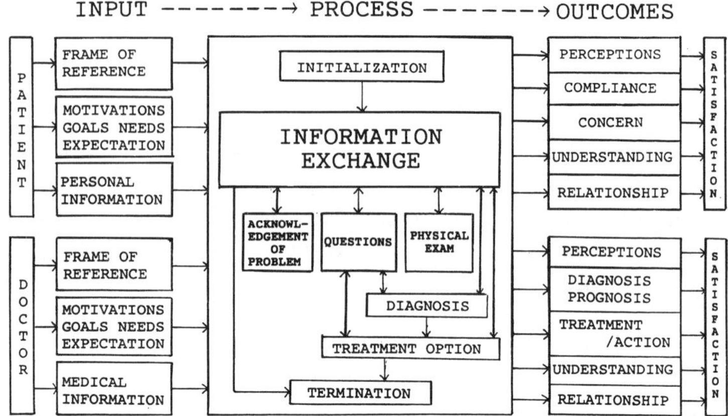

Figure 1.4 A model of doctor–patient communication. Source: Frederikson (1992)

behind the events they experience. The principal theoretical framework has been a collection of models together known as attribution theory (Heider, 1958; Jones and Davis, 1965; Kelley, 1967), which propose that people are 'intuitive scientists', whose task is to decide whether a given occurrence was caused by the person or by environmental circumstances, and whether the causes are stable or changeable. They may also try to decide whether the causes are controllable or beyond human influence (Weiner, 1985, 1986, 1992). At the heart of attribution processes lies the notion of control, and our purpose in this section of the chapter is to examine the way in which concepts of control have influenced social psychological thinking about health behaviours and outcomes.

Locus of control

The first concept to appear historically was *locus* of control (Rotter, 1966), whose roots were to be found both in attribution theory and in Rotter's own social learning theory of reinforcement. Rotter argued that individuals had a 'generalized expectancy or belief' in internal or external control of their reinforcements.

A single dimension was sufficient to account for variability from person to person, individual differences were relatively stable over time and circumstances, and locus of control was best seen as a component of personality.

The implications of the concept for *health* behaviour and outcomes have subsequently been explored by a number of groups (see the reviews by Lefcourt, 1976; Strickland, 1978; and Wallston *et al.*, 1987, for example), of whom the most influential has been Wallston and his colleagues. Wallston argues that perceived control is best defined as a belief that one 'can determine one's own internal status and behaviour, influence one's environment, and/or bring about desired outcomes' (Wallston *et al.*, 1987). Wallston's own Multi-Dimensional Health Locus of Control scale (Wallston, Wallston and De Vellis, 1978) proposes three orthogonal dimensions: internal, powerful others and chance. Powerful others might be doctors, for example, or employers, or influential members of the family, and a given behaviour or outcome might be seen as under the control of any or all of the dimensions. I might, for example, consider that my ill health is attributable to my own behaviour, my employer's failure to protect me and/or chance, but my car accident I shall probably blame on the person with whom I collided – the powerful other. The model allows more subtle and complex judgements to be made than was possible with Rotter's scheme, and it acknowledges that individuals may vary according to the behaviour, circumstance or outcome in question.

Locus of control has been used to account for findings in a wide range of health behaviours and outcomes, including smoking, birth control, weight loss, preventive health behaviours, sick role behaviours and adherence to health care advice and treatment regimens (Wallston and Wallston, 1978). What emerges most strongly from the research, however, is that, whereas locus of control began as a *perceptual* index, the literature has moved on to incorporate behavioural or *actual* control over environmental contingencies or events, and also *need* for control (Steptoe, 1989). At the same time, a variety of related concepts has evolved, all to do with personal control, but varying in whether perception, behaviour or need are their focus: self-efficacy (Bandura, 1977, 1982; O'Leary, 1985); learned helplessness (Seligman, 1975; Abramson, Seligman and Teasdale, 1978; Burns and Seligman, 1989); explanatory style (Kamen and Seligman, 1987); dispositional optimism (Scheier and Carver, 1985, 1987); controllability (Glass and Singer, 1972; Sherrod, 1974); predictability (Cohen, 1988); desire for control (Burger, 1985); sense of control (Schulz, 1976; Rodin and Langer, 1977; Rodin, 1986); powerlessness (Bauman and Udry, 1972); hardiness (Kobasa, 1982); and competence (Libassi and Maluccio, 1986).

Among the most interesting research has been a series of attempts at intervention, designed to measure the effects upon health of manipulating the environment to increase actual control – or at least the feeling and possibility of actual control. Syme, for example, is working with bus drivers, to give them greater control over their timetables (Ragland *et al.*, 1987; Winkleby, Ragland and Syme, 1988); and Wallston has been working on the way in which barium meals are administered (Wallston *et al.*, 1987) and what can be done to reduce nausea after chemotherapy for cancer, and discomfort and malaise after surgery (Wallston, 1989). The classic intervention study, however, was by Rodin and Langer (1977).

Rodin and Langer studied residents in an old people's home, and found that they had little control over their day-to-day lives, because the staff took over all responsibility. An experiment was set up to explore the possibilities of change, and residents were assigned at random to an experimental group (N = 47) or a comparison group (N = 44). In the experimental condition the administrator of the home gave a talk to the group, in which the residents' responsibility for themselves was emphasized, while the comparison group were given a talk that stressed the staff's responsibility for the residents. To reinforce the talk, the experimental residents were given plants to look after and water, while the comparison group were given plants to be tended by the staff. Eighteen months after the intervention began, the experimental residents were found to be significantly more 'actively interested' than the others, and more 'sociable', 'self-initiating', 'vigorous' and almost but not quite significantly 'happier'. Most striking of all, significantly fewer of the experimental group had died – seven against thirteen. The manipulation had been simple, and apparently very small, but the benefits were enormous. Similar findings, on control over when visitors were allowed to call, were published at the same time by

Schulz (1976), and the Rodin and Langer study was subsequently replicated by Pohl and Fuller (1980).

Explanatory style

Explanatory style is the way people habitually explain the causes of good or bad events, and recent evidence indicates that it has important effects on people's susceptibility to illness. The origins of the construct are to be found in learned helplessness and attribution theories. Experiments by Seligman (1975) indicated that organisms exposed to uncontrollable aversive events began to behave as if they were helpless. They showed motivational, cognitive and emotional deficits which are thought to be *learned* (Seligman and Maier, 1967; Hiroto and Seligman, 1975; Maier and Seligman, 1976). The motivational deficits were lower response initiation (passivity), the cognitive deficits involved failure to learn new response-outcome contingencies, and the emotional deficits involved loss of self-esteem. Seligman and his colleagues incorporated these observations into a learned helplessness theory of depression, but three theoretical difficulties emerged with the theory. First, it did not specify when and why someone might experience emotional deficits with a loss of self-esteem following an uncontrollable aversive event and when not. Second, it could not account for the chronicity or time course of the deficits: sometimes they were short and at other times they were long-lasting. Third, it failed to account for the generality of the motivational and cognitive deficits produced by helplessness: under some conditions they were cross-situational, while under others they were situation-specific.

The theoretical difficulties were addressed by Abramson *et al.* (1978) in a reformulation of learned helplessness theory along attributional lines. The authors argued that 'when a person finds he is helpless, he asks *why* he is helpless' (*ibid.*, p. 50). Three dimensions, each corresponding to the three theoretical difficulties we have mentioned, are relevant in arriving at an explanation. If the events are seen as caused by something about the individual (internal attributions) as opposed to something about the situation (external attributions), then the helplessness deficits will lead to loss of self-esteem. If the uncontrollable event is attributed to non-transient factors (stable attributions) rather than transient ones (unstable attributions), the deficits will be long-lasting, and finally, if the events are attributed to causes present in a variety of situations (global attributions) rather than few (specific attributions) the deficits will be generalized to other situations. In summary, Abramson *et al.* argued that people who habitually explain bad events by internal, stable and global causes and good events by external, unstable and specific causes – the pessimistic explanatory style, as they called it – will be more likely to experience general and lasting helplessness deficits with self-esteem loss than people with an 'optimistic' style. People who explain the causes of bad events in this way expect them to be uncontrollable and to occur consistently over time and in different situations. They are therefore hopeless as to changing the future and behave passively when change occurs. A pessimistic explanatory style predisposes the individual to depression. The theory has also appeared in another reformulation as hopelessness theory (Abramson, Metalsky and Alloy, 1989), and recently Kamen and Seligman (1987) have extended the range of deficits, claiming that pessimistic explanatory style also leads to increased morbidity.

There have been two main techniques for measuring explanatory style. The first is called the Content Analysis of Verbatim Explanations (CAVE) and makes use of verbatim written or spoken material by the subject that provides causal explanations for events (diaries, letters, essays, speeches). The explanation of the event is rated by three independent judges on seven-point scales according to internality, stability and globality, and so provides an explanatory style profile which can be used to predict later outcomes (Peterson and Seligman, 1986). In one particularly interesting study, the technique was used to explore whether pessimistic rumination on the part of American presidential candidates would predict their defeat (Zullow and Seligman, 1990). The authors claimed a causal association, but there were a number of, sometimes amusing, critiques of their method (Scheier and Carver, 1990; Simonton, 1990; Tetlock, 1990).

The second technique for measuring explanatory style is the Attributional Style Questionnaire, which is a 48-item self-report instrument (Peterson *et al.*, 1982). The questionnaire was designed to measure an individual's characteristic style across a variety of situations and consists of twelve hypothetical events, six positive and six negative. Subjects are asked to imagine each event happening to them and to assign a cause to each one. Causes are then rated for internality, stability and globality. Findings from the technique suggest that explanatory style influences a variety of health outcomes, including infectious diseases, health status, lowered immunocompetence and poor health (Kamen and Seligman, 1987; Peterson and Seligman, 1987; Peterson, 1988; Peterson, Seligman and Vaillant, 1988; Lin and Peterson, 1990; Kamen-Siegel *et al.*, 1991). The possible mechanisms include reduced competence of the immune system in people with a pessimistic style, and poor self-care, self-help and response to challenge.

Type A behaviour pattern (TABP)

Earlier, we pointed to the distinction between perceived control, actual control and need for control. TABP belongs to the last of those categories, and emerged as a concept from the work of Rosenman in the mid-1970s. Friedman and Rosenman (1974), using their Structured Interview, identified a pattern of behaviour that categorized people who were 'involved in an aggressive and incessant struggle to achieve more and more in less and less time' (Friedman and Rosenman, 1974). The major components were 'competitive striving for achievement, impatience and a sense of urgency, aggression, and easily aroused hostility' (Booth-Kewley and Friedman, 1987). The significance of TABP was that it appeared from prospective evidence to predict coronary heart disease (CHD) (Rosenman *et al.*, 1975), but the literature soon developed a sense of scepticism. There were two main questions: were all the components of TABP implicated in CHD; and was it chronic heart disease, acute heart attack or fatal heart attack that was predicted?

The Structured Interview (Rosenman, 1978) asked people about their characteristic way of responding to situations that potentially elicit impatience, competitiveness and hostility. The interviewer scored both the content of what was said and the way in which it was said, including vocal speed, explosiveness and volume. Although there is little evidence that the measures reflect the respondent's everyday pattern of behaviour, or indeed that the Structured Interview and other measures of TABP correlate (Matthews, 1982) – the Jenkins Activity Survey (Jenkins, Zyzanski and Rosenman, 1971, 1978), the Framingham

Questionnaire (Haynes *et al.*, 1978) and the Bortner Questionnaire (Bortner, 1969) – nevertheless, many studies have been published, and the data have now been subjected to a meta-analysis (Booth-Kewley and Friedman, 1987). Booth-Kewley and Friedman drew three main conclusions: TABP showed a modest but reliable relationship with CHD; the size of the relationship was similar for all CHD outcomes, whether morbidity or mortality; and depression produced as strong a relationship with CHD as did TABP, with anger/hostility/aggression and anxiety close behind. Overall, it was concluded,

> the picture of the coronary-prone personality emerging from this review does not appear to be that of the workaholic, hurried, impatient individual, which is probably the image most frequently associated with coronary proneness. Rather, the true picture seems to be one of a person with one or more negative emotions: perhaps someone who is depressed, aggressively competitive, easily frustrated, anxious, angry, or some combination. (Booth-Kewley and Friedman, 1987, p. 358)

One of the difficulties with meta-analysis is to know quite what to include, and an important reservation in the Booth-Kewley and Friedman paper was that prospective studies generally produced weaker relationships than cross-sectional studies. Another author, Matthews, therefore went on to conduct a further analysis in which cross-sectional data were excluded (Matthews, 1988). She also introduced stringent additional criteria: high-risk studies were to be separated from population studies; each set of results was to be weighted by the number of subjects; and 'negative emotions' were to be analysed separately from TABP. As in Booth-Kewley and Friedman, there were three main conclusions, but they were very different: Type A was *not* a reliable predictor of the incidence of CHD; when a relationship did emerge, it was generally with *initial* CHD events, not CHD events overall; and *hostility* rather than depression was the best predictor among the so-called 'negative emotions'.

For the non-specialist reader (and writer), the debate is sometimes technical and difficult to follow, but it provides a salutary warning about the consequences of rushing to conclusions when concepts have not been properly defined and refined, when there is no agreement about measurement or about the appropriate outcomes to monitor, and when there are differences of opinion about how to design and conduct satisfactory studies. For the time being, the last word is with Friedman and Booth-Kewley: 'All in all, there is a remarkable degree of consensus about what we know and what we need to know. Strong evidence emerges that Type A behavior (assessed by the Structured Interview) is a significant risk factor for coronary heart disease, but the Type A construct still has not been adequately defined' (Friedman and Booth-Kewley, 1988, p. 381).

Cognitive dispositions: beliefs and attitudes

Like perceived control, beliefs and attitudes are best regarded as cognitive dispositions, aspects of the individual's habitual way of viewing the world that predispose to particular ways of coping and behaving. An attitude is a summary statement of one's overall stance with respect to an object or behaviour. I am 'in favour of' vegetables, for example, but 'against' fat, and 'pro' swimming but 'anti' jogging. Attitudes to objects are often consistent with attitudes to related behaviours, though not always, and the expectation is that attitudes will *predict* behaviour. Whether or not they do has been a central issue in social psychology for many years, from Allport onwards (Allport, 1935), and it is the one that concerns us in this section of the chapter. There are two main theoretical approaches to consider: the Health Belief Model (Rosenstock, 1974; Janz and Becker, 1984); and the Theory of Reasoned Action (Fishbein and Ajzen, 1975).

The Health Belief Model

The Health Belief Model appeared in the 1950s and was published in its full form in Rosenstock (1974). It began as an attempt to understand people's failures to take up preventive and screening programmes then on offer in the United States, and it was soon applied to how people responded when they were ill and whether they complied with treatment and advice. The model belongs to the expectancy-value tradition of theories, which argues that behaviour is dependent on two main variables: the value an individual places on a particular goal; and the individual's estimate of the likelihood that a given action will achieve that goal. Applied to health, the variables become the desire to avoid illness (or to recover from it if one is ill already), and the belief that given illnesses will be prevented (or overcome) by given behaviours.

The model is constructed from three dimensions: perceived susceptibility or vulnerability; perceived severity; and perceived benefits and barriers (Figure 1.5). Imagine that we are trying to predict which of a group of men will take up jogging in the hope of preventing coronary heart disease. Perceived susceptibility refers to how much at risk of coronary heart disease the individual believes himself to be, for whatever reason. Perceived severity is about how serious an effect on his life he believes the disease would have, both medically and socially. Perceived benefits and barriers refer to the perceived rewards and costs of doing the behaviour – for example, the short-term relaxation and enjoyment of jogging and the long-term benefits to health, against the short-term costs of time and energy and the possible

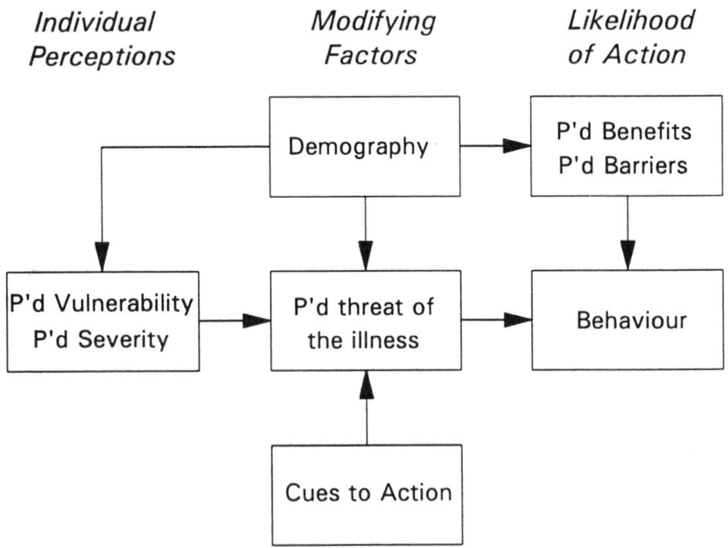

Figure 1.5 Health Belief Model.

long-term harm to tendons and joints. For the illness to be perceived as sufficiently threatening for action to be precipitated at all, there will probably be some 'cue to action', whether internal (perhaps the beginnings of symptoms of disease) or external (perhaps a mass media campaign). Perceived susceptibility and vulnerability create the threat, probably in combination with a cue to action, demographic variables may 'moderate' the threat (to use the model's terms), and perceived benefits and barriers will come into play at the end, when the threat has been recognized and the individual is on the point of taking action.

An enormous volume of research on the model has been conducted, and a detailed review was published by Janz and Becker (1984). Since then there have been many studies on, for example, AIDS prevention (reviewed by Hayes, 1991); self-examination for breast cancer (for example, Ronis and Harel, 1989; Champion, 1990); attendance for dental checks (for example, Chen and Land, 1986, 1990); attendance for cervical smears (for example, Hennig and Knowles, 1990); and attendance for routine medical checks (for example, Norman and Fitter, 1991). The largest category, as the examples suggest, continues to be research on *preventive* health behaviours and, in general, the strongest support for the model has come from prospective studies, in which behaviour is measured sometime *after* the measurement of beliefs. The leading predictor of behaviour has most commonly been perceived barriers, which means that the people most likely to take up the preventive behaviour are those who see the costs as minimal. Perceived susceptibility is often a stronger predictor than perceived benefits – even though most people apparently see themselves as relatively invulnerable to almost all diseases, a condition known as 'unrealistic optimism' (Weinstein, 1980, 1982). The weakest predictor of behaviour in the Health Belief Model has generally been perceived severity, because people are relatively unthreatened by negative long-term outcomes, which are unlikely to happen and are difficult to imagine.

The Theory of Reasoned Action

The Theory of Reasoned Action has wider applicability than the Health Belief Model because it is about beliefs and attitudes in general and is not specific to health. It is another example of the expectancy-value approach, and it arose out of dissatisfaction with the concept of attitude as it stood in the literature in the early 1970s. The traditional definition of attitude included three components – cognition, affect and intention – and the literature was in turmoil because attitudes defined in that way appeared not to predict behaviour reliably, even though theory said they should (Wicker, 1969). The reason, argued Fishbein and Ajzen, lay in the conceptual ambiguity of the definition, and the solution was simply to separate the components. The cognitive component became 'belief' in the Theory or Reasoned Action, and 'attitude' was reserved for affect. The foundation of the model was thus cognition, and behaviour was seen as the outcome of reasoned information processing. The immediate determinant of behaviour was intention, intention was a function of attitude, and attitude was derived from component beliefs (Figure 1.6).

To predict behaviour from the Theory of Reasoned Action, one must first measure the individual's beliefs, of which there are two sets of interest: personal beliefs and normative beliefs. Imagine that we are concerned with jogging again, this time whether I will take it up myself. My personal beliefs are about what I see as the consequences – for example, helping to prevent coronary heart disease, helping to cure my asthma, helping me to lose weight – each of which I see as positive or negative and more or less likely to be the case. My normative beliefs are my perceptions of what people who are important to me want me to

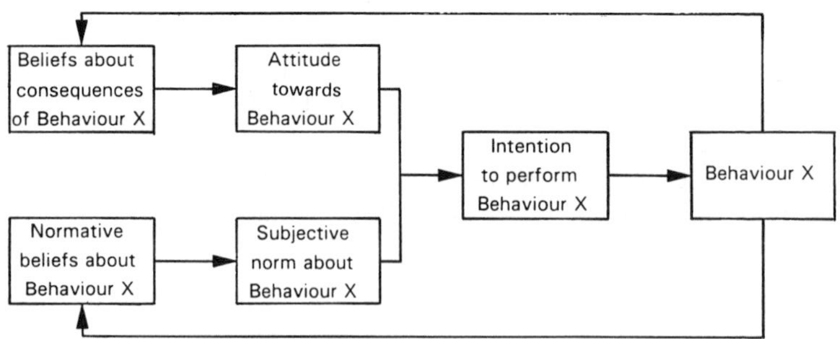

Figure 1.6 Theory of Reasoned Action. Source: Fishbein and Ajzen (1975)

do – whether my wife wants me to take up jogging, my children, my doctor, and so on. From the combination of my personal beliefs we can infer whether I am broadly in favour of taking up jogging or broadly against it, and it is that 'summary statement' that for Fishbein and Ajzen is attitude. The corresponding summary of my normative beliefs is subjective norm. Attitude and subjective norm together underpin my intention, and from my intention comes my behaviour.

Like the Health Belief Model, the Theory of Reasoned Action has generated a great deal of research, and useful reviews of the literature on many areas, including health, are to be found in Ajzen and Fishbein (1980), Canary and Siebold (1984), Sheppard, Hartwick and Warshaw (1988), Ajzen (1988, 1991) and Tesser and Shaffer (1990). Three main conclusions emerge: first, attitudes do predict behaviour, and a large proportion of the variance is often explained; second, personal beliefs and attitude are generally better predictors than normative beliefs and subjective norm; and third, behaviour is predicted less well by attitudes to objects than by attitudes to related behaviours. There is, however, one important limitation to the model, namely that it applies only to behaviour that is perceived to be under the individual's control. If, for example, I have a positive attitude towards attending a clinic for a new screening service, but I cannot read the appointment card or I have no means of transport, the model will apparently *fail* to predict my intentions and behaviour. What was missing was an estimate of what Bandura called self-efficacy – 'the conviction that one can execute the behaviour required to produce the outcomes' (Bandura, 1977) – and a revised version of the model was needed.

The new model, the Theory of Planned Behaviour, was published by Ajzen (1988). Personal beliefs and normative beliefs are measured as before, and so are attitude and subjective norm, but people are now asked to say how much control they believe they have over executing the intention in question. Perceived behavioural control, as Ajzen called it, is placed alongside attitude and subjective norm in the model, and is said to lead to behaviour indirectly, through the mediation of intention, and perhaps directly too. Even within an individual, perceived behavioural control will vary from behaviour to behaviour and from circumstance to circumstance – unlike Rotter's perceived locus of control, for example, which is a stable disposition – and it reflects both internal factors, such as perceived skill and ability, and external factors, such as encouragements and obstacles. It is thus the individual's estimate of the 'presence or absence of requisite resources and opportunities' (Ajzen, 1991, p. 196). The Theory of Planned Behaviour has already been used in a variety of studies on health – including Schifter and Ajzen (1985) on weight loss, Godin, Vezina and Leclerc (1989) on taking exercise after giving birth, Beale and Manstead (1991) on limiting infants' sugar intake, and Otis, Godin and Lambert (in press) on using condoms – and there is good evidence that perceived behavioural control predicts intention. Whether there is also a *direct* path to behaviour, however, remains uncertain, since only Schifter and Ajzen (1985) have so far included a measure of behaviour in their analysis.

The models compared

There are a number of important points of comparison to make between the Health Belief Model and the Theory of Reasoned Action, and we shall draw attention to ten in particular. First, both models are expectancy-value models, in which a central influence on behaviour is the way it is perceived. In the Health Belief Model the main consideration is perceived benefits and barriers, and in the Theory of Reasoned Action it is expected outcomes. Second, the Health Belief Model, unlike the Theory of Reasoned Action, allows beliefs about the *object* of the behaviour to play a part – perceived susceptibility to the illness and its perceived consequences – as well as beliefs about the behaviour. For Fishbein and Ajzen, beliefs about objects are ruled out on both conceptual and empirical grounds: what influences whether I smoke is not whether I like cigarettes but whether I like *smoking* cigarettes. Third, there is no explicit role for cues to action in the Theory of Reasoned Action, though implicitly they may be seen as colouring one's beliefs about behaviour – witnessing a friend's injuries from a road accident may influence my beliefs about my driving, for example. Fourth, there is no explicit role for normative pressure in the Health Belief Model, though it could perhaps be seen as part of perceived benefits and barriers and even cues to action – a nagging family, for example. Fifth, neither model acknowledges the role of efficacy beliefs to the extent of incorporating them formally, though the Theory of Planned Behaviour, of course, does.

The sixth point of comparison between the Health Belief Model and the Theory of Reasoned Action is that neither allows a direct route from previous behaviour to current behaviour. The Health Belief Model says nothing about what has been done in the past, while the Theory of Reasoned Action argues that any effect of previous behaviour is taken up by *current beliefs*. The issue still awaits empirical resolution (Bentler and Speckart, 1979; Ajzen, 1991). Seventh, both traditions accept that, if people do not value their health or think about it actively, behaviour will not be predicted successfully. Eighth, where beliefs come from, their origins in socialization and experience, plays no part in the models; all that matters is *what* the beliefs are. Ninth, both approaches have important implications for intervention – through health education, for example – and indeed, a welcome new direction for the literature to take would be to develop prospective research in which the effects of interventions are monitored over time. Finally, there are very different roles in the two models for what we have called social inputs. The Health Belief Model allows that demographic variables may 'moderate' beliefs, but Fishbein and Ajzen, like ourselves, argue for *mediation*: demographic and other social inputs influence beliefs and attitudes, which in turn lead on to intentions and behaviour. Prospective analyses, in which causal pathways between variables can be properly mapped out over time, seem to us to be essential if the full significance of beliefs and attitudes is to be understood and issues such as the role of previous behaviour are to be settled. As yet, there is little published research of that sort.

Stress and coping

Stress is a subjective experience which is a threat to the quality of life and to physical and psychological well-being (Krantz,

Grunberg and Baum, 1985). The outcomes or symptoms of stress may be physical, psychological or behavioural. Stress has been implicated in the causation of many disorders, including cardiovascular and respiratory disorders, metabolic malfunction, cancer, and psychosomatic and psychiatric illness. Because the emotional and physical strain that accompanies stress is uncomfortable, people are motivated to do things to reduce it, a process called coping. The purpose of this section of the chapter is to outline the main theoretical approaches to stress and coping, and to examine the implications for health outcome.

Approaches to the study of stress

There have been three main approaches to the study of stress. The first sees stress as the *stimulus* characteristics of negative or disturbing environments (Symonds, 1947; Weitz, 1970). Events or circumstances that are perceived as threatening, producing feelings of tension or arousal, are called *stressors*. Researchers typically study the impact of natural disasters such as earthquakes or floods, severe life-events such as bereavement, or daily hassles.

The second approach sees stress as a *response*, and focuses on people's reactions to stressors (Selye, 1956; Levi, 1974). There are two related components: a psychological component which involves cognitions, emotions and behaviour, and a physiological component which involves heightened bodily arousal. A person's response to a stressor is called *strain*.

In the third approach, which has probably been the most influential, stress is seen as a *process* which involves continuous interactions and adjustments – called *transactions* – between the person and the environment (Lazarus, 1966; Folkman, Schaefer and Lazarus, 1979). Stress is now seen not just as a stimulus or a response, but as a set of processes in which the person is an active agent, able to influence the impact of stressors through emotional, cognitive and behavioural strategies. Lazarus defines stress as 'the psychological state which derives from people's appraisals of their adaptation to the demands which are made of them' (Lazarus, 1966). It is thus the condition that results when person–environment transactions lead people to perceive a discrepancy between the demands of a situation and their resources or ability to cope with those demands (Lazarus, 1966; Folkman and Lazarus, 1985). The absolute magnitude of demands is not the most important factor that determines the experience of symptoms of stress, for there may be significant individual differences in the stress experienced by people faced with the same demands, because of differences in ability to cope.

A transactional model of coping: Folkman and Lazarus (1985)

The most influential of the transactional approaches has been that of Folkman and Lazarus (1985). A central feature of the model (Figure 1.7) is the process of *cognitive appraisal* (Lazarus, 1966), a mental process by which people assess whether a demand threatens their well-being and appraise their resources for meeting it. There are two components: primary and secondary appraisal. When a potentially stressful event occurs, people attempt to assess its meaning and its likely impact on their well-being. Primary appraisal yields a judgement of the event as irrelevant, benign-positive or stressful, and events appraised as stressful receive further appraisal for three implications: harm-loss, threat and challenge. Harm-loss refers to the amount of damage that has occurred already, threat is the expectation of future harm, and challenge is the opportunity to achieve growth and mastery.

After primary appraisal, secondary appraisal begins – though the two processes may sometimes occur almost simultaneously and feed back into each other (Cohen and Lazarus, 1983). Secondary appraisal is a cognitive assessment of the resources available for coping, and the formulation of a response to the stressor. The person asks: what can I do about this event, what resources can I use, and what will the outcome be? Coping resources are 'aspects of the individual's external and internal environment which are either directly or completely under the individual's control; they exist in a quiescent state ready to mediate in a positive or negative direction the individual's response to the advent of a stressor' (Shapiro, 1983). They may be physical, material, social, psychological or intellectual, and the nature and type of coping generated by people will be determined by the coping resources in their environment.

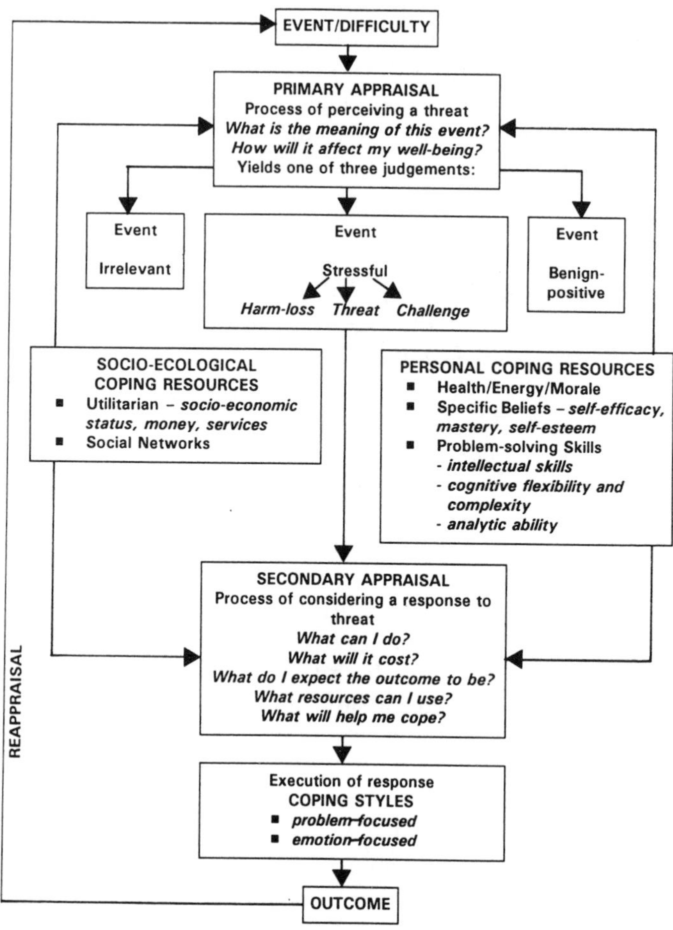

Figure 1.7 The Lazarus–Folkman model of stress and coping

According to Folkman, Shaefer and Lazarus (1979), there are five categories of coping resources: *utilitarian resources*, including socio-economic status, money, available services; *health, energy or morale*, including pre-existing physical and psychiatric illness, depression; *social networks*, including close interpersonal relationships; *general and specific beliefs*, including self-efficacy, mastery, self-esteem; and *problem-solving skills*, including intellectual skills, cognitive flexibility and complexity, and analytic ability.

Coping is thus a problem-solving process by which people try to manage the perceived discrepancy between the demands made on them in a stressful situation and their resources for meeting it. Coping efforts can be directed towards the threat itself or towards the emotional distress caused by the threat (Lazarus, Averill and Opton, 1974). In most discussions in the literature, it is assumed that coping is an organized activity and that 'coping strategies' are employed, whether cognitive or behavioural: for example, expressing emotions, beginning a new activity, thinking about the problem, or asking for help. Failure to cope carries no negative connotations: demands may simply exceed resources.

The research evidence

To study the coping process, Lazarus and his colleagues developed a measure called Ways of Coping (Folkman and Lazarus, 1980, 1985), which consists of a series of statements about possible coping strategies individuals may or may not use. Respondents are asked to say which they do use and which they do not. A distinction between two general styles of coping is embedded in the scale. The first, problem-focused coping, consists of problem-solving or carrying out some thought or action to reduce or ameliorate the source of stress. The second, emotion-focused coping, consists of reducing or managing the emotional distress caused by the event. Folkman and Lazarus (1980) have noted that, although most stressors elicit both types of coping, emotion-focused coping tends to be used when people feel that the stressor is something that must be endured, while problem-focused coping is used when they feel that something constructive can be done. Research typically finds, however, that responses to the Ways of Coping scale form more than two factors (Felton, Revenson and Hinrichsen, 1984; Vitaliano *et al.*, 1985; Folkman *et al.*, 1986; Aldwin and Revenson, 1987; MacCarthy and Brown, 1989). There are now many coping scales and many typologies of coping (Rosentiel and Keefe, 1983; Brown and Nicassio, 1987; Namir *et al.*, 1987; Carver, Scheier and Weintraub, 1989; Endler and Parker, 1990; Rolide *et al.*,

1990). The major issues at present in the literature are whether individuals use the same coping strategies across situations or whether they select a specific coping response depending on the stressor (Pearlin and Schooler, 1978; McFarlane *et al.*, 1983) and whether certain coping responses are consistently better than others. Overall, coping methods involving avoidance appear to be as effective as those involving active attention, but *active* attention strategies are associated with better adjustment in the long term (see the meta analysis by Suls and Fletcher, 1985).

One of the more interesting studies of coping styles comes from Greer, Morris and Pettingale (1979), who conducted a prospective five-year study of 69 female patients with early breast cancer. Patients' psychological responses to the diagnosis of cancer were assessed three months post-operatively. When responses were related to outcome five years after the operation, recurrence-free survival was found to be significantly more common among patients who had initially reacted with denial or with a fighting spirit than among patients who had responded with stoic acceptance or feelings of helplessness and hopelessness. Further follow-up after ten years confirmed the finding (Pettingale *et al.*, 1985). The same authors later replicated their study in a larger sample of 178 patients, including Hodgkin's disease and non-Hodgkin's lymphoma, and similar results emerged (Burgess, Morris and Pettingale, 1988).

A second study comes from Brown and Nicassio (1987). The study made use of the Vanderbilt Pain Management Inventory, which assesses the frequency with which pain patients use active or passive coping strategies when their pain reaches a greater level of intensity. Active coping was found to be associated with reports of less pain, less depression, less functional impairment and higher general self-efficacy. Passive coping was related to reports of greater depression, greater pain and flare-up activity, greater functional impairment and lower self-efficacy.

A third study, an empirical test of Folkman and Lazarus's model (Folkman, Schaefer and Lazarus, 1979), was carried out by Quine and Pahl (1991). A total of 166 mothers of children with severe learning disabilities were studied, and a measure of stress was taken by means of a 24-item inventory of physical and psychological symptoms. A stepwise hierarchical multiple regression analysis was carried out in which the variables were entered in blocks reflecting their assumed causal priority. The first block contained the stressor variables – characteristics of the child such as age, academic skill scores and behaviour problem score. The second block contained coping resources from the five categories outlined by Folkman and Lazarus. The third block contained coping strategies. The results of the analysis showed that the stressor variables accounted for 12 per cent of the variance, while four of the five coping resource variables added a further 43 per cent to the explained variance. Each variable entered into the analysis explained a significant proportion of additional variance, and altogether 55 per cent of the variance in stress scores was explained. None of the coping strategy variables made a significant contribution.

As to *how* coping has its effects on health outcome, Cohen and Lazarus (1979) have suggested several possible mechanisms. Coping has been shown to affect hormone levels, to cause direct effects on tissues, and to impinge on the immune system (Kielcolt-Glaser *et al.*, 1987). Interpersonal coping styles may influence the type of care received (demanding patients may have their complaints dealt with more quickly). Jensen (1987), for example, found that cancer patients who coped by complaining and expressing high levels of negative affect survived longest. In contrast, positive coping, 'fighting spirit', may have positive physiological consequences, as we saw in the work of Greer, Morris and Pettingale. Effective coping may also lead to quicker recovery from illness. Active coping strategies appear to be particularly effective (Brown and Nicassio, 1987).

Appropriate and inappropriate behaviours

We come now to the final set of mediators between inputs and outcomes, namely behaviours. We divide behaviours into two sets, appropriate and inappropriate. Appropriate behaviours are those that promote and maintain health and help to prevent illness – taking exercise and eating a healthy diet, for example, and taking up preventive health services such as dental care and health screening. Inappropriate behaviours are those that damage health – drug and alcohol abuse, smoking, and so on. Of all the behaviours, cigarette smoking has received much the most attention because of its established association with morbidity and mortality (Doll and Peto, 1981; Froggatt, 1988), and it therefore provides the focus for this section of the chapter.

The prevalence of smoking

In most of the developed world, the proportion of people who smoke has fallen steadily since the late 1960s. The decline has been greatest in men: more than half the adult male population were regular smokers in the late 1960s, but by the late 1980s the proportion was down to a third. Among women, the trend has been less clear but the proportion of women who smoke is generally smaller than the proportion of men, though the difference is sometimes very slight (Marsh, 1987).

In Britain, the most detailed information comes from the General Household Survey conducted by OPCS, and the most recent findings are for 1990 (OPCS, 1991c). Figure 1.8 shows that

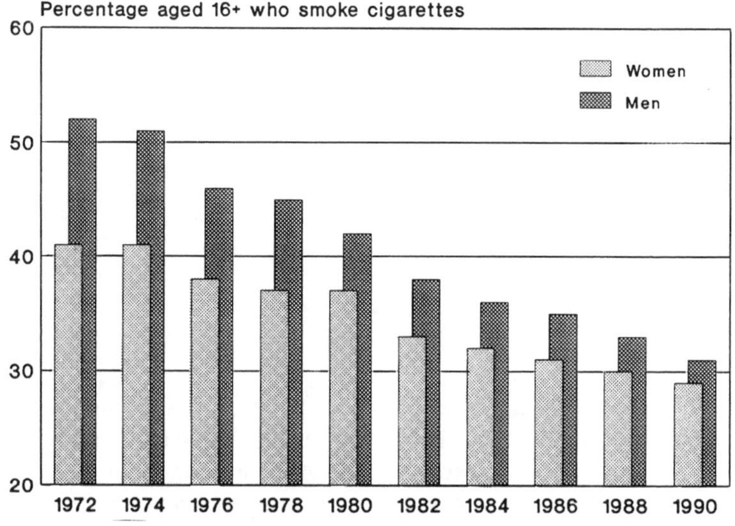

Figure 1.8 Cigarette smoking by sex: 1972–90. Source: OPCS General Household Survey

31 per cent of men aged 16 and over and 29 per cent of women are now regular smokers – one cigarette or more a day for a year – compared with 52 per cent for men in 1972 when the General Household Survey began and 41 per cent for women. The gap between men and women has closed in recent years, and indeed, among 16–19 year olds, the figure is now higher for women than men – 32 per cent against 28 per cent. Data from secondary school children in 1990 also show a higher prevalence among females than males (Lader and Matheson, 1991). Smoking is strongly related to social class, with the lowest prevalence in professional occupations and the highest in unskilled manual occupations, and the difference between the sexes is greatest among working-class people. Men smoke more cigarettes a week than women, 118 on average for all smokers against 97, and fewer men than women smoke low tar brands. In total, British adults smoke over 70 billion cigarettes a year.

The consequences of smoking

The classic study of what smoking does to health was conducted by Doll and Peto (1976). In October 1951, a questionnaire was sent to all male doctors whose names were on the British *Medical Register* and who were believed to be resident in the United Kingdom. The questionnaire asked a few simple questions about the doctors' smoking habits, and replies were received from 34,440, a response rate of 69 per cent. From the records of what is now OPCS, every death among the sample was noted from November 1951 to October 1971. Further questionnaires were sent to survivors in 1957, 1966 and 1972, to monitor changes in smoking, and the response rates were 98.4 per cent, 96.4 per cent, and 97.9 per cent. The study was thus prospective, large scale and on a sample of people who were strongly motivated to take part.

The analysis of the data addressed three main questions: how would mortality ratios in regular smokers and life-long non-smokers compare; what would be the principal causes of death, the diseases from which smokers and non-smokers died; and how significant would be the number of cigarettes smoked. The findings were stark. First, when age-specific mortality ratios were examined, the rate for smokers under 70 was approximately 2:1 compared with non-smokers, and for those over 70 it was 1.5:1 (there were fewer smokers left to die). Second, for the sample as a whole, the causes of death with the most marked differences were chronic bronchitis and emphysema (16:1 for smokers against non-smokers) and lung cancer (10:1). Eight other diseases, however, also produced significant differences: cancer of the oesophagus, of non-specified respiratory sites, and of the rectum; respiratory tuberculosis; pulmonary heart disease; and ischaemic heart disease, myocardial degeneration and aortic aneurism. In other words, the respiratory system, the cardiovascular system and even the digestive system were all implicated. Third, there was a clear relationship with the number of cigarettes smoked each day. The mortality ratios against non-smokers for lung cancer, for example, were 5:1 for people who smoked 1–14 cigarettes a day, 10:1 for 15–24 a day, and 22:1 for 25 or more a day. For chronic bronchitis and emphysema, the pattern was stronger still: 12:1, 16:1 and 29:1. For every one of the causes of death that had distinguished smokers from non-smokers, there was a significant trend with the number of cigarettes smoked – and a similar trend was present for many other causes of death that had *not* distinguished smokers from non-smokers. Thus, smoking led to premature death, it killed by a variety of means, and the greater the number of cigarettes smoked each day, the greater the risk.

Large-scale prospective studies are, of course, difficult and expensive to mount. The largest in progress at the moment is being conducted by the American Cancer Society with more than one million subjects (Garfinkel, 1985), and one of the preliminary outcomes of the study has been a recent attempt, by Peto and his colleagues, to estimate the *worldwide* consequences of smoking (Peto *et al.*, 1992). The initial analyses of the American data show age-specific mortality ratios more than double those for non-smokers – as in Doll and Peto (1976) – and the inference is that around half the deaths among American smokers are caused by tobacco. By extrapolation from the data, using conservative statistical analyses of published international mortality figures (WHO, 1987), Peto has estimated that around two million people are dying of smoking each year in the developed world, giving a figure of approximately 20 million in the decade

1990–9: five or six million in the European Community, five or six million in the United States, five million in the former USSR, three million in Eastern Europe and European countries not in the European Community; and two million elsewhere (Australia, Canada, Japan and New Zealand combined). More than half the deaths are to people aged 35–69, which makes tobacco the largest single cause of premature death. On current smoking patterns, Peto estimates, over 20 per cent of people now living in the developed world will eventually be killed by smoking – ¼ billion out of a current total of just under 1¼ billion. All these are figures for the *developed* world, it should be remembered; what is happening, and will happen, in the *developing* world is not yet known.

Smoking and the young

For theory and for policy and practice alike, perhaps the most important questions to ask about smoking are when and why do young people start (Royal College of Physicians, 1992). The most detailed data on 'when' come from the OPCS study by Lader and Matheson (1991), which we have mentioned already. Around 10,000 secondary school children in England, Scotland and Wales were interviewed about their smoking habits in 1990 and were asked to keep a diary. Over the whole age range studied, 11–15, roughly 10 per cent were regular smokers (defined as one or more cigarettes a week) and 6 per cent smoked occasionally. By the age of 15, the figures were 25 per cent and 10 per cent, which suggests that the majority of people who are regular smokers in adulthood are already well established in their smoking careers before they leave school. Of the regular smokers aged 11–15, around 30 per cent smoked 10 or more cigarettes a day, and 65 per cent expected to continue smoking when they left school. More than 15 per cent of the boys in the sample and 10 per cent of the girls had tried a cigarette by the age of 11 – some as early as 6 – and the figures for those who were now regular smokers were more than 35 per cent for boys and 25 per cent for girls. The estimated consumption of cigarettes among 11–15 year olds in England, Scotland and Wales combined is now almost 20 million cigarettes a week.

As to why children take up smoking, Lader and Matheson were able to provide some interesting clues from the children's backgrounds. First, regular smoking was much more common among children whose siblings were smokers than among those whose siblings were not: 28 per cent for boys and 29 per cent for girls, against 6 per cent and 6 per cent. Second, there was a similar association with parental smoking: when both parents were smokers, 13 per cent of boys and 17 per cent of girls smoked regularly, but when neither was a smoker the figures were 5 per cent and 6 per cent. Third, smoking was associated with drinking: 43 per cent of regular smokers drank once or more a week, against only 5 per cent of non-smokers. What seemed to be implied by the data was thus a pattern of normative values among 'smoking families' which distinguished them from 'non-smoking families' – but, since the data were cross-sectional and retrospective, it was impossible to attribute cause and effect. For that, prospective data would be needed.

A number of prospective studies do now exist in both the United States and Britain (see the reviews by McNeil *et al.*, 1988; Eiser *et al.*, 1989; and Goddard, 1990), and one of the most extensive from Britain is a study by McNeil *et al.* (1988). Over 2,100 secondary school children aged 11–13, all of them non-smokers at the time, were approached in 1983 (Nelson *et al.*, 1985). They completed a lengthy questionnaire on their background, beliefs, attitudes and behaviour, and 30 months later they were followed up and asked whether they had taken up smoking in the meantime. Some 35 per cent of them had – though a number said they had already given up – and the critical question was whether the Time 1 measures would predict the change in behaviour. The data were examined by multivariate analysis, and one predictor stood out: children who had taken up smoking at some time during the 30 months were over four times more likely to have tried smoking by Time 1 than those who were still non-smokers. Beliefs and attitudes played little if any part – even the normative values suggested by the data of Lader and Matheson – but significant contributions were made by sex (being female), uncertainty about future smoking intentions, the experience of having been drunk at least once in the past, having a boyfriend or girlfriend, believing that teachers and friends 'would not mind' if one took up smoking, and attending a school at which many of the teachers were smokers. A child with the 'least favourable' combination of factors was over 14 times more likely to have taken up smoking than a child with the 'most favourable' combination. The implications were clear: the best predictor of behaviour was *prior* behaviour; and the best way to discourage smoking was to prevent the first puff.

Social inputs, social psychological mediators and health outcomes: a theoretical model

The purpose of our book, as we said at the beginning of the chapter, is to examine the social psychological mechanisms by which social inputs are turned into outcomes, and to trace the pathways of causality. We have discussed definitions of health, described what we mean by social inputs, and reviewed the social psychological factors and processes that may act as mediators between inputs and health outcomes. Now we present a model to try to draw together the relationships (see Figure 1.9).

The effect of social inputs on health is mediated by two sets of variables, we argue, socio-emotional and cognitive. Socio-emotional variables are shown in the top branch of the model and cognitive variables in the lower branch. *Socio-emotional* variables include people's experience of severe life-events and difficulties,

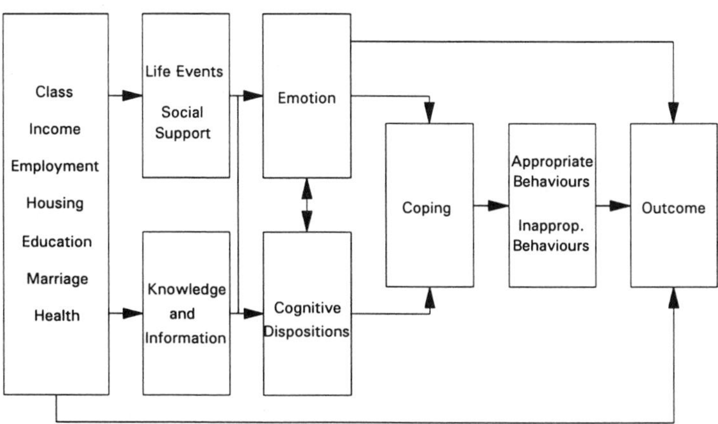

Figure 1.9 A model of mediators in health

and the availability and adequacy of supportive relationships offering cognitive guidance, tangible assistance, emotional support, social reinforcement and opportunities for socializing. Severe life-events, in combination with low social support, we argue, will lead to emotional problems, including loss of self-esteem, anxiety and depression. *Cognitive* variables include people's access to information, and knowledge, and their cognitive dispositions. By cognitive dispositions, as we have seen, we mean personal control and beliefs and attitudes, both of which we see as products of information, knowledge and communication.

The core of our model is coping. Coping is to do with how people confront the stresses in their lives, and we argue that the resources and strategies they have available – and the way they select and implement them – are products of both the socio-emotional and cognitive levels of our model. For example, someone who lacks social support and is already weakened by adversity may have fewer coping strategies to call upon than someone who is free from adversity and has access to supportive relationships, and the particular strategies selected may differ too. Again, someone with an optimistic explanatory style, who focuses on external, unstable and specific explanations for life's difficulties, may display different coping patterns from someone with a pessimistic style, who expects bad events to occur consistently and to be uncontrollable, and who reacts with helplessness, depression and passivity whenever they do occur. Socio-emotional and cognitive problems may act separately or in combination, and will result in coping styles and strategies characterized by helplessness or hopelessness, altered perceptions of risk and vulnerability, and an undue willingness to behave in risky ways, by smoking in pregnancy or driving when drunk, for example. From dysfunctional coping styles come inappropriate behaviours, and from inappropriate behaviours it is a small step to negative health outcomes.

The model we have outlined is at present essentially a framework for integrating past findings and guiding future research, for there are many gaps to be filled in the existing body of knowledge, and much to be done to establish the strengths and weights of the proposed links and causal pathways. There are several points of caution to make. First, we do not wish to argue that all links between social inputs and health outcomes are mediated in the way the model emphasizes. There may well be direct links between some of the social inputs and health outcomes, or links through behaviour that bypass social psychological mechanisms. We acknowledge the possibility of other links, and we do not wish to argue in an either/or way. Second, as we have noted, there are methodological weaknesses in parts of the research, and we have tried to weight our discussion accordingly. Sometimes, indeed, there are straightforward gaps in what is known about the relationships between social inputs and social psychological factors, and the issues remain to be resolved. Finally, we acknowledge that the model is oversimplified, but the oversimplification is deliberate because we have had dual purposes: to integrate the existing literature theoretically and to point to directions for future research. Only a few of the variables that are known to be important have been included, and the causal pathways are all seen as left-to-right with no allowance for feedback loops. As we hope we have made clear throughout the discussion, our main concern has been to draw attention to the social psychological mechanisms by which social inputs influence health outcomes, and that is why we have kept our model as simple as possible.

In the next three chapters we shall present our own research, on pregnancy outcome, breast cancer screening, and motorcycling. Though the three areas may seem to be very different, the common theme is our concern to explore the role of social psychological factors as mediators between social inputs and health outcomes. It is that concern, and the opportunities the areas give us to test aspects of our model, that binds the research together. In our work on pregnancy, the main outcomes will be satisfaction with medical communications and with the birth experience, and the principal mediators will be knowledge and attitudes. In the chapter on breast cancer, our focus will be attendance for screening and satisfaction with the service, and the extent to which attitudes and expectations about the process are predictors. In the research on motorcycling, we shall examine safe and unsafe riding behaviours and their relationship with accidents, and we shall explore how far behaviour can be predicted from attitudes. In the final chapter of the book, the themes that emerge from our findings will be brought together, and we shall discuss their implications for theory and for policy and practice.

References

Abramson L Y, Metalsky G I and Alloy L B (1989), Hopelessness depression: a theory based subtype of depression, *Psychological Review*, 96, 358–72.

Abramson L Y, Seligman M E P and Teasdale J D (1978), Learned helplessness in humans: critique and reformulation, *Journal of Abnormal Psychology*, 87, 49–74.

Ajzen I (1988), *Attitudes, Personality, and Behavior*, Chicago: Dorsey Press.

Ajzen I (1991), The Theory of Planned Behavior, *Organizational Behavior and Human Decision Processes*, 50, 179–211.

Ajzen I and Fishbein M (1980), *Understanding Attitudes and Predicting Social Behavior*, Englewood Cliffs, NJ: Prentice Hall.

Aldwin C and Revenson T A (1987), Does coping help? A re-examination of the relation between coping and mental health, *Journal of Personality and Social Psychology*, 53, 337–48.

Allgulander C and Lavori P W (1991), Excess mortality among 3302 patients with 'pure' anxiety neurosis, *Archives of General Psychiatry*, 48, 599–602.

Alloway R and Bebbington P (1987), The buffer theory of social support – a review of the literature, *Psychological Medicine*, 17, 91–108.

Allport G W (1935), Attitudes. In C Murchinson (Ed.), *A Handbook of Social Psychology*, 798–844, Worcester, Mass: Clark University Press.

Anderson K O and Masur F (1983), Psychological preparation for invasive medical and dental procedures, *Journal of Behavioral Medicine*, 6, 1–40.

Bandura A (1977), Self-efficacy: toward a unifying theory of behavioral change, *Psychological Review*, 84, 191–215.

Bandura A (1982), Self-efficacy mechanisms in human agency, *American Psychologists*, 37, 122–47.

Bauman K E and Udry J R (1972), Powerlessness and regularity of contraception in an urban Negro male sample: a research note, *Journal of Marriage and the Family*, 34, 112–14.

Beale D A and Manstead A S R (1991), Predicting mothers' intentions to limit frequency of infants' sugar intake: testing the theory of planned behavior, *Journal of Applied Social Psychology*, 21, 409–31.

Bebbington P (1985), Psychosocial aetiology of schizophrenia and affective disorders. In M Michaels (Ed.), *Psychiatry*, Philadelphia: Lippincot.

Bentler P M and Speckart G (1979), Models of attitude–behavior relations, *Psychological Review*, 86, 452–64.

Berkman L F (1984), Assessing the physical health effects of social networks and support, *Review of Public Health*, 5, 413–32.

Berkman L F (1986), Social networks, support and health: taking the next step forward, *American Journal of Epidemiology*, 123, 559–62.

Berkman L F and Syme S L (1979), Social networks, host resistance, and mortality: a nine-year follow-up study of Alemada County residents, *American Journal of Epidemiology*, 109, 186–204.

Black D (1980), *Inequalities in Health* (Black Report), Report of a research working group chaired by Sir Douglas Black, London: DHSS.

Black D W, Warrack G and Winokur G (1985), The Iowa record-linkage study I, Suicides and accidental deaths, *Archives of General Psychiatry*, 42, 71–83.

Blane D, Smith G D and Bartley M (1990), Social class differences in years of potential life lost: size, trends, and principal causes, *British Medical Journal*, 301, 429–32.

Booth-Kewley S and Friedman H S (1987), Psychological predictors of heart disease: a quantitative review, *Psychological Bulletin*, 101, 3, 343–62.

Bortner A (1969), A short rating scale as a potential measure of pattern A behavior, *Journal of Chronic Disease*, 22, 87–91.

Boyle C M (1970), Differences between patients' and doctors' interpretations of common medical terms, *British Medical Journal*, 2, 286–89.

British Medical Association (1987), Deprivation and ill-health, *BMA Discussion Paper*, London: BMA.

Broadhead W E, Kaplan B H, Sherman A J, Wagner E H, Schoenback V J, Grimson R, Heyden S, Tibblin G and Gehlbach S H (1983), The epidemiologic evidence for a relationship between social support and health, *American Journal of Epidemiology*, 117, 521–37.

Brown G W (1974), Meaning, measurement and stress of life-events. In B S Dohrenwend and B P Dohrenwend (Eds.), *Stressful Life-events: Their Nature and Effects*, 217–43, New York: Wiley.

Brown G W (1987), Social factors and the development and course of depressive disorders in women: a review of a research programme, *British Journal of Social Work*, 17, 615–34.

Brown G and Nicassio P (1987), Development of a questionnaire for the assessment of active and passive coping strategies in chronic pain patients, *Pain*, 31, 53–64.

Brown G W, Andrews B, Harris T, Adler Z and Bridge L (1986a), Social support, self-esteem and depression, *Psychological Medicine*, 16, 813–31.

Brown G W, Bhrolcháin M N and Harris T (1975), Social class and psychiatric disturbance among women in an urban population, *Sociology*, 9, 225–54.

Brown G W, Bifulco A, Harris T and Bridge L (1986b), Life stress, chronic subclinical symptoms and vulnerability to clinical depression, *Journal of Affective Disorders*, 11, 1–9.

Brown G W, Andrews B, Harris T, Adler Z and Bridge L (1986c), Social support, self-esteem and depression, *Psychological Medicine*, 16, 813–31.

Brown G W and Birley J L T (1968), Crises and life changes and the onset of schizophrenia, *Journal of Health and Social Behaviour*, 9, 203–14.

Brown G W and Harris T (1978), *Social Origins of Depression: A Study of Psychiatric Disorder in Women*, London: Tavistock.

Bruce M L and Leaf P (1989), Psychiatric disorders and 15-month mortality in a community sample of older adults, *American Journal of Public Health*, 79, 727–30.

Burger J (1985), Desire for control and achievement-related behaviors, *Journal of Personality and Social Psychology*, 48, 1520–33.

Burgess C, Morris T and Pettingale K (1988), Psychological response to cancer diagnosis. II Evidence for coping styles, *Journal of Psychosomatic Research*, 32, 263–72.

Burns M and Seligman M E P (1989), Explanatory style across the life span: evidence for stability over 52 years, *Journal of Personality and Social Psychology*, 56, 471–77.

Canary D J and Siebold D R (1984), *Attitudes and Behavior: An Annotated Bibliography*, New York: Praeger.

Cartwright A (1967), *Patients and Their Doctors*, London: Routledge & Kegan Paul.

Cartwright A and Anderson R (1981), *General Practice Revisited*, London: Tavistock.

Carver C S, Scheier M F and Weintraub J K (1989), Assessing coping strategies: a theoretically based approach, *Journal of Personality and Social Psychology*, 56, 267–83.

Casadebaig F and Quemada N (1989), Mortality in psychiatric inpatients, *Acta Psychiatrica Scandinavica*, 79, 257–63.

Cassel J (1976), The contribution of the social environment to host resistance, *American Journal of Epidemiology*, 104, 107–23.

Champion V L (1990), Breast self-examination in women 35 and older: a prospective study, *Journal of Behavioral Medicine*, 13, 523–38.

Chen M and Land K C (1986), Testing the Health Belief Model: LISREL analysis of alternative models of causal relationships between health beliefs and preventive dental behavior, *Social Psychology Quarterly*, 49, 56–60.

Chen M and Land K C (1990), Socioeconomic status (SES) and the Health Belief Model: LISREL analysis of unidimensional versus multidimensional formulations, *Journal of Social Behavior and Personality*, 5, 263–84.

Cleary P J (1980), A checklist for life-events research, *Journal of Psychosomatic Research*, 24, 199–207.

Cline D W and Chosey J J (1972), A prospective study of life changes and subsequent health changes, *Archives of General Psychiatry*, 27, 51–3.

Cobb S (1976), Social support as a moderator of life stress, *Psychosomatic Medicine*, 38, 300–14.

Cohen C and Sokolovsky J (1978), Schizophrenia and social networks, *Schizophrenia Bulletin*, 4, 546–60.

Cohen F and Lazarus R S (1979), Coping with the stress of illness. In C G C Stone, F Cohen and N E Adler (Eds.), *Health Psychology: A Handbook*, San Francisco: Jossey-Bass.

Cohen F and Lazarus R S (1983), Coping and adaptation in health and illness. In D Mechanic, *Handbook of Health, Health Care and the Health Professions*, New York: Free Press.

Cohen S (1988), Aftereffects of stress on human performance and social behavior, *Psychological Bulletin*, 88, 82–108.

Cohen S and McKay G (1984), Social support, stress and the buffering hypothesis: a theoretical analysis. In A Baum, J E Singer and S E Taylor (Eds.), *Handbook of Psychology*, Hillsdale, NJ: Erlbaum.

Cohen S L and Hajioff J (1972), Life events and the onset of acute closed-angle glaucoma, *Journal of Psychosomatic Research*, 16, 335–41.

Cole R (1979), The understanding of medical terminology used in printed health education materials, *Health Education Journal*, 38, 111–21.

Connolly J (1976), Life events before myocardial infarction, *Journal of Human Stress*, 2, 3–17.

Coryell W H (1988), Panic disorder and mortality, *Psychiatric Clinics of North America*, 11, 433–40.

Coryell W, Noyes R and Clancy J (1982), Excess mortality in panic disorder: a comparison with primary unipolar depression, *Archives of General Psychiatry*, 39, 701–3.

Coryell W, Noyes R and House J D (1986), Mortality among outpatients with anxiety disorders, *American Journal of Psychiatry*, 143, 508–10.

Creed F H (1981), Life events and appendicectomy, *Lancet*, 1381–5.
Creed F H (1985), Life events and physical illness, *Journal of Psychosomatic Research*, 29, 113–23.
Day R, Nielsen J A, Korten A and Ernberg G (1987), Stressful life events preceding the acute onset of schizophrenia: a cross-national study from the World Health Organization, *Culture, Medicine and Psychiatry*, 11, 123–205.
Dean A and Lin N (1977), The stress-buffering role of social support: problems and prospects for systematic investigation, *Journal of Nervous and Mental Disease*, 165, 6, 403–17.
Department of Health (1991), *The Health of the Nation: A Consultative Document for Health in England*, London: HMSO.
Devine E C and Cook T D (1982), A meta-analysis of the effects of psycho-educational interventions on length of postsurgical hospital stay, *Nursing Research*, 32, 267–74.
Doak L G and Doak C C (1980), Patient comprehension profiles: recent findings and strategies, *Patient Counselling and Health Education*, 2, 101–6.
Dohrenwend B P and Dohrenwend B S (1981), Socioenvironmental factors, stress and psychopathology, *American Journal of Community Psychology*, 9, 124–64.
Dohrenwend B S and Dohrenwend B P (1978), Some issues in research on stressful life events, *Journal of Nervous and Mental Diseases*, 106, 7–15.
Dohrenwend B S, Krasnoff L, Askenasy A A and Dohrenwend B P (1978), Exemplification of a method for scaling life events: the Peri Life Events Scale, *Journal of Health and Social Behaviour*, 19, 205–29.
Doll R and Peto R (1976), Mortality in relation to smoking: 20 years' observations on male British doctors, *British Medical Journal*, 2, 1525–36.
Doll R and Peto R (1981), *The Causes of Cancer*, Oxford/New York: Oxford University Press.
Eiser J R, Morgan M, Gammage P and Gray E (1989), Adolescent smoking: attitudes, norms and parental influence, *British Journal of Social Psychology*, 28, 193–202.
Elbourne D and Oakley A (1990), An overview of trials of social support during pregnancy: effects on gestational age at delivery and birthweight. In H W Berendes, W Kessel and S Yaffe (Eds.), *Advances in the Prevention of Low Birthweight*, New York: Perinatology Press.
Endler N S and Parker D A (1990), The multidimensional assessment of coping: a critical evaluation, *Journal of Personality and Social Psychology*, 58, 844–54.

Felton B J, Revenson T A and Hinrichsen G A (1984), Stress and coping in the explanation of psychological adjustment among chronically ill adults, *Social Science and Medicine*, 18, 889–98.

Finlay-Jones R A (1988), Life events and psychiatric illness. In A S Henderson and G D Burrows (Eds.), *Handbook of Social Psychiatry*, Amsterdam: Elsevier.

Fishbein M and Ajzen I (1975), *Belief, Attitude, Intention and Behavior*, Reading, Mass: Addison-Wesley.

Flesch R (1948), A new readability yardstick, *Journal of Applied Psychology*, 32, 221–33.

Flint C and Poulengeris P (1987), *Know Your Midwife*, London: Heinemann.

Folkman S and Lazarus R S (1980), An analysis of coping in a middle aged community sample, *Journal of Health and Social Behaviour*, 21, 219–39.

Folkman S and Lazarus R S (1985), If it changes it must be a process: a study of emotion and coping during three stages of a college examination, *Journal of Personality and Social Psychiatry*, 48, 150–70.

Folkman S, Lazarus R S, Dunkel-Schelter C, Delongis A and Gruen R J (1986), Dynamics of a stressful encounter. Cognitive appraisal, coping and encounter outcomes, *Journal of Personality and Social Psychology*, 50, 992–1003.

Folkman S, Schaefer C and Lazarus R (1979), Cognitive processes as mediators of stress and coping. In V Hamilton and D Warburton (Eds.), *Human Stress and Cognition: An Information Processing Approach*, London: Wiley.

Frederikson L G (1992), Development of an integrative model for medical communication, *Health Communication*, in press.

Fredman L, Schoenbach V J, Kaplan B H, Blazer D G, James S H, Kleinbaum D G and Yankaskas B (1989), The association between depressive symptoms and mortality among older participants in the Epidemiologic Catchment Area in Piedmont Health Survey, *Journal of Gerontology*, 44, 149–56.

Friedman H S and Booth-Kewley S (1988), Validity of the Type A construct: a reprise, *Psychological Bulletin*, 104, 381–4.

Friedman H S and Rosenman R H (1974), *Type A Behavior and Your Heart*, New York: Knopf.

Froggatt P (1988), *Fourth Report of the Independent Scientific Committee on Smoking and Health*, London: HMSO.

Funch D P, Marshall J R and Gebhardt G P (1986), Assessment of a short scale to measure social support, *Social Science and Medicine*, 23, 3, 337–44.

Garfinkel L (1985), Selection, follow-up and analysis in the American Cancer Society prospective studies. In L Garfinkel, O Ochs and M Mushinksi (Eds.), *Selection, Follow-up and Analysis in Prospective Studies: A Workshop*, NCI Monograph 67, National Cancer Institute, NIH Publication No 85–2713, 1985; 49–52.

Glass D C and Singer J E (1972), *Urban Stress: Experiments on Noise and Social Stressors*, New York: Academic Press.

Goddard E (1990), *Why Children Start Smoking*, London: HMSO.

Godin G, Vezina L and Leclerc O (1989), Factors influencing intentions of pregnant women to exercise after giving birth, *Public Health Reports*, 104, 188–95.

Goldberg E L and Comstock G W (1976), Life events and subsequent illness, *American Journal of Epidemiology*, 104, 146–53.

Goldberg E L, Comstock G W and Hornstra R K (1979), Depressed mood and subsequent physical illness, *American Journal of Psychiatry*, 136, 530–4.

Goldblatt P (1989), Mortality by social class, 1971–85, *Population Trends*, 56, 6–15.

Goldblatt P (Ed.) (1990), *Longitudinal Study: Mortality and Social Organization*, London: HMSO.

Gore S (1981), Stress buffering functions of social support: an appraisal and clarification of research models. In B S Dohrenwend and B P Dohrenwend (Eds.), *Stressful Life Events and Their Contexts*, New York: Prodist.

Greenblatt M, Becerra R M and Serafetinides E A (1982), Social networks and mental health: an overview, *American Journal of Psychiatry*, 139, 8, 977–84.

Greer S, Morris T and Pettingale K (1979), Psychological response to breast cancer: effect on outcome, *Lancet*, ii, 785–7.

Guze S B and Robins E (1970), Suicide and primary affective disorders, *British Journal of Psychiatry*, 117, 437–42.

Hadlow J and Pitts M (1991), The understanding of common health terms by doctors, nurses and patients, *Social Science and Medicine*, 32, 193–6.

Hart N (1987), Class, health and survival: the gap widens, *Radical Community Medicine*, Spring 10.

Hayes J A (1991), Psychological barriers to behavior change in preventing human immunodeficiency virus (HIV) infection, *Counselling Psychologist*, 19, 585–602.

Haynes S G, Feinleib M, Levine S, Scotch N and Kannel W B (1978), The relationship of psychosocial factors to coronary heart disease in the Framingham Study II. Prevalence of coronary heart disease, *American Journal of Epidemiology*, 107, 384–402.

Health Promotion and Research Trust (1987), *The Health and Lifestyle Survey*, Cambridge: HPRT.

Heider F (1958), *The Psychology of Interpersonal Relations*, New York: Wiley

Heisel S J (1972), Life changes as etiologic factors in juvenile rheumatoid arthritis, *Journal of Psychosomatic Research*, 16, 411–20.

Henderson A S (1980), Personal networks and the schizophrenias, *Australia and New Zealand Journal of Psychiatry*, 14, 255–9.

Henderson A S (1984), Interpreting the evidence on social support, *Social Psychiatry*, 19, 49–52.

Henderson A S and Brown G W (1988), Social support: the hypothesis and the evidence. In A S Henderson and G D Burrows (Eds.), *Handbook of Social Psychiatry*, Amsterdam: Elsevier.

Henderson A S, Byrne D G and Duncan-Jones P (1981), *Neurosis and the Social Environment*, Sydney: Academic Press.

Henderson A S, Byrne D G, Duncan-Jones P, Adcock S, Scott R and Steele G P (1978a), Social bonds in the epidemiology of neurosis: a preliminary communication, *British Journal of Psychiatry*, 132, 463–6.

Henderson A S, Duncan-Jones P, McAuley H and Ritchie K (1978b), The patient's primary group, *British Journal of Psychiatry*, 132, 74–86.

Henderson A S, Duncan-Jones P, Byrne D G and Scott R (1980), Measuring social relationships: the interview schedule for social interaction, *Psychological Medicine*, 10, 723–34.

Hennig P and Knowles A (1990), Factors influencing women over 40 years to take precautions against cervical cancer, *Journal of Applied Social Psychology*, 20, 1612–21.

Hinde R A (1979), *Towards Understanding Relationships*, London: Academic Press.

Hinkle L E and Wolff H G (1957), The nature of man's adaptation to his total environment and the relation of this to illness, *Archives of Internal Medicine*, 99, 442–60.

Hiroto D S and Seligman M E P (1975), Generality of learned helplessness in man, *Journal of Personality and Social Psychology*, 31, 311–27.

Holmes T H, Hawkins N S, Bowerman C E, Clarke E P Jr and Joffe J R (1957), Psychosocial and psychophysiological studies of tuberculosis, *Psychosomatic Medicine*, 19, 134–43.

Holmes T H and Masuda M (1974), Life change and illness susceptibility. In B S Dohrenwend and B P Dohrenwend (Eds.), *Stressful Life Events: Their Nature and Effects*, 45–72, New York: Wiley.

Holmes T H and Rahe R H (1967), The Social Readjustment Rating Scale, *Journal of Psychosomatic Research*, 11, 213–18.

House J S (1981), *Work Stress and Social Support*, Reading, Mass: Addison-Wesley.

Illsley R (1980), *Professional or Public Health: Sociology in Health and Medicine*, London: Nuffield Provincial Hospitals Trust.

Illsley R (1986), Occupational class, selection and the production of inequalities in health, *Quarterly Journal of Social Affairs, 2*, 151–65.

Illsley R and LeGrand J (1987), The measurement of inequality, LSE Welfare State Programme: Discussion Paper No. 12, London: LSE.

Janz N K and Becker M H (1984), The Health Belief Model: a decade later, *Health Education Quarterly*, 11, 1–47.

Jenkins C D, Zyzanski S J and Rosenman R H (1971), Progress toward validation of a computer-scored test for the Type A coronary-prone behavior pattern, *Psychosomatic Medicine*, 33, 193–202.

Jenkins C D, Zyzanski S J and Rosenman R H (1978), Coronary-prone behavior: one pattern or several?, *Psychosomatic Medicine*, 40, 25–43.

Jensen M R (1987), Psychological factors predicting the course of breast cancer, *Journal of Personality*, 55, 317–42.

Jones E E and Davis K E (1965), From acts to dispositions: the attribution process in person perception. In L Berkowitz (Ed.), *Advances in Experimental Social Psychology*, Vol. 2, 219–66, New York: Academic Press.

Kahn R L and Antonucci T C (1980), Convoys over the life course: attachment, roles and social support, *Life Span Development and Behavior*, 3, 253–86.

Kamen L P and Seligman M E P (1987), Explanatory style and health, *Current Psychology Research and Reviews*, 6, 207–18.

Kamen-Siegel L, Rodin J, Seligman M E and Dwyer J (1991), Explanatory style and cell-mediated immunity in elderly men and women, *Health Psychology*, 10, 229–35.

Kanner A D, Coyne J C, Schaefer C and Lazarus R S (1981), Comparison of two modes of stress measurement: daily hassles and uplifts versus major life events, *Journal of Behavioral Medicine*, 4, 1–39.

Kaplan B H (1991), Social psychology of the immune system: a conceptual framework and review of the literature, *Social Science and Medicine*, 33, 909–23.

Kaplan B H, Cassel J C and Gore S (1977), Social support and health, *Medical Care*, 15, 5, Suppl, 47–58.

Keehn R J, Goldberg I D and Beebe G W (1974), Twenty-four year mortality follow-up of army veterans with disability separations for psychoneurosis in 1944, *Psychosomatic Medicine*, 36, 27–46.

Kelley H H (1967), Attribution theory in social psychology. In D Levine

(Ed.), *Nebraska Symposium on Motivation*, Lincoln: University of Nebraska Press.

Kielcolt-Glaser J K, Fisher L D, Ogrocki P, Stout J, Speicher C E and Glaser R (1987), Marital quality, marital disruption and immune function, *Psychosomatic Medicine*, 49, 13–34.

Kincey J A, Bradshaw P W and Ley P (1975), Patients' satisfaction and reported acceptance of advice in general practice, *Journal of the Royal College of General Practitioners*, 25, 558–66.

Klaus M H, Kennell J H, Robertson S S and Sosa R (1986), Effects of social support during parturition on maternal and infant morbidity, *British Medical Journal*, 293, 585–7.

Kobasa S C (1982), The hardy personality: Toward a social psychology of stress and health. In G S Sanders and J Suls (Eds.), *Social Psychology of Health and Illness*, Hillsdale, NJ: Erlbaum.

Korsch B M (1989), The past and future of research in doctor–patient relations. In M Stewart and D Roter (Eds.), *Communicating with Medical Patients*, 246–51, London: Sage.

Korsch B M, Gozzi E and Francis V (1968), Gaps in doctor–patient communication. I: Doctor–patient interaction and patient satisfaction, *Pediatrics*, 42, 855–71.

Korsch B M and Negrete V (1972), Doctor–patient communication, *Scientific American*, August, 66–73.

Krantz D S, Grunberg W E and Baum A (1985), Health psychology, *Annual Review of Psychology*, 26, 91–8.

Lader D and Matheson J (1991), *Smoking among Secondary School Children in 1990*, London: HMSO.

Lazarus R S (1966), *Psychological Stress and the Coping Process*, New York: McGraw-Hill.

Lazarus R S (1984), Puzzles in the study of daily hassles, *Journal of Behavioral Medicine*, 7, 375–89.

Lazarus R S, Averill J R and Opton E M (1974), The psychology of coping: issues of research and assessment. In G V Coehio, D A Hamburg and J E Adams (Eds.), *Coping and Adaptation*, New York: Basic Books.

Lefcourt H (1976), *Locus of Control*, Hillsdale, NJ: Erlbaum.

LeGrand J (1985), Inequalities in health: the human capital approach, LSE Welfare State Programme Discussion Paper No. 1, London: LSE.

LeGrand J (1986), Inequalities in health and health care: a research agenda. In R G Wilkinson (Ed.), *Class and Health*, London: Tavistock, 115–25.

Lei H and Skinner H S (1980), A psychosometric study of life events and social readjustment, *Journal of Psychosomatic Research*, 24, 57–66.

Leighton D C, Harding J S, Macklin D B, Hughes C C and Leighton A

H (1963), Psychiatric findings of the Stirling County Study, *American Journal of Psychiatry*, 119, 1021–6.

Levi L (1974), Stress, distress and psychosocial stimuli. In A McLean (Ed.), *Occupational Stress*, Springfield, Ill.: Charles C Thomas.

Ley P (1977), Psychological studies of doctor-patient communication. In S Rachmann (Ed.) *Contributions to Medical Psychology*, Vol. 1, Oxford: Pergamon.

Ley P (1988), *Communicating with Patients*, London: Chapman & Hall.

Ley P, Bradshaw P W, Kincey J and Atherton S T (1976), Increasing patients' satisfaction with communication, *British Journal of Sociology and Clinical Psychology*, 15, 217–20.

Ley P and Spelman M (1967), *Communicating with the Patient*, London: Staples Press.

Libassi M F and Maluccio A (1986), Competence-centred social work: prevention in action, *Journal of Primary Prevention*, 6, 168–80.

Lieberman A A and Coburn A F (1986), The health of the chronically mentally ill: a review of the literature, *Community Mental Health*, 22, 104–11.

Lin E H and Peterson C (1990), Pessimistic explanatory style and response to illness, *Behaviour Research and Therapy*, 28, 243–8.

Lin N and Dean A (1984), Social support and depression: a panel study, *Social Psychiatry*, 19, 83–91.

Linder-Pelz S (1982), Social psychological determinants of patient satisfaction: a test of five hypotheses, *Social Science and Medicine*, 16, 583–9.

Litwak E and Szelenyi I (1969), Primary group structures and their functions: kin, neighbors and friends, *American Sociological Review*, 34, 465–81.

Lowenthal M F (1964), Social isolation and mental illness in old age, *American Sociological Review*, 29, 54–70.

Lynch J (1977), *The Broken Heart. The Medical Consequences of Loneliness*, New York: Basic.

MacCarthy B and Brown R (1989), Psychosocial factors in Parkinson's disease, *British Journal of Clinical Psychology*, 28, 41–52.

Macintyre S (1986), The patterning of health by social position in contemporary Britain: directions for sociological research, *Social Science and Medicine*, 23, 393–415.

Macintyre S (1988), A review of the social patterning and significance of measures of height, weight, blood pressure and respiratory function, *Social Science and Medicine*, 27, 327–37.

Maguire P and Faulkner A (1988a), Communicate with cancer patients: 1 Handling bad news and difficult questions, *British Medical Journal*, 297, 907–9.

Maguire P and Faulkner A (1988b), Communicate with cancer patients: 2 Handling uncertainty, collusion and denial, *British Medical Journal*, 297, 972–4.

Maier S F and Seligman M E P (1976), Learned helplessness: theory and evidence, *Journal of Experimental Psychology: General*, 105, 3–46.

Markush R E (1977), Mortality and community mental health: the Alachua County, Florida mortality study, *Archives of General Psychiatry*, 34, 1393–401.

Marmot M G (1986), Social inequalities in mortality: the social environment. In R G Wilkinson (Ed.), *Class and Health*, London: Tavistock, 21–33.

Marmot M G and McDowall M E (1986), Mortality decline and widening social inequalities, *Lancet*, 2 August, 274–6.

Marmot M G, Shipley M J and Rose G (1984), Inequalities in death – specific explanations of a general pattern?, *Lancet*, 5 May, 1003–6.

Marsh A (1987), *The Dying of the Light*, Copenhagen: WHO Regional Committee for Europe.

Maslow A H (1968), *Toward a Psychology of Being*, New York: Van Nostrand.

Mathews A and Ridgeway V (1984), Psychological preparation for surgery. In A Mathews and A Steptoe (Eds.), *Health Care and Human Behaviour*, London: Academic Press.

Matthews K A (1982), Psychological perspective on the Type A behavior pattern, *Psychological Bulletin*, 81, 293–323.

Matthews K A (1988), Coronary heart disease and Type A behaviors: update on and alternative to the Booth-Kewley and Friedman (1987) quantitative review, *Psychological Bulletin*, 104, 373–80.

Mazzuca S A (1982), Does patient education in chronic disease have therapeutic value?, *Journal of Chronic Diseases*, 35, 521–9.

McFarlane A H, Norman G R, Steiner D and Roy R G (1983), The process of social stress: stable, reciprocal and mediating relationships, *Journal of Health and Social Behaviour*, 24, 160–73.

McNeil A D, Jarvis M J, Stapleton J A, Russell M A H, Eiser J R, Gammage P and Gray E M (1988), Prospective study of factors predicting uptake of smoking in adolescents, *Journal of Epidemiology and Community Health*, 43, 72–8.

Monroe S M (1983), Social support and disorder: toward an untangling of cause and effect, *American Journal of Community Psychology*, 11, 1, 81–97.

Mueller D P (1980), Social networks: a promising direction for research on the relationship of the social environment to psychiatric disorder, *Social Science and Medicine*, 14, 147–61.

Mullen P D, Green L W and Persinger G S (1985), Clinical trials of patient education for chronic conditions: a comparative meta-analysis of intervention types, *Preventive Medicine*, 14, 753–81.

Murphy J M (1990), Depression in the community: findings from the Sterling County Study, *Canadian Journal of Psychiatry*, 35, 390–2.

Murphy J M, Manson R R, Olivier D C, Sobol A M and Leighton A H (1987), Affective disorders and mortality, *Archives of General Psychiatry*, 44, 473–80.

Murphy J M, Manson R R, Olivier D C, Sobol A M and Leighton A H (1989), Mortality risk and psychiatric disorders: results of a general physician survey, *Social Psychology and Psychiatric Epidemiology*, 24, 134–42.

Namir S, Wolcott D L, Fawzy F I and Alumbaugh M J (1987), Coping with AIDS: psychological and health implications, *Journal of Applied Social Psychology*, 17, 309–28.

Nelson S C, Budd R J, Morgan M J, Gammage P and Gray E (1985), The Avon prevalence study: a survey of cigarette smoking in secondary schoolchildren, *Health Education Journal*, 44, 12–15.

Nielsen J, Homma A and Biorn-Henriksen T (1977), Follow-up fifteen years after geronto-psychiatric prevalence study, *Journal of Gerontology*, 5, 554–61.

Norman P and Fitter M (1991), Predicting attendance at health screening: organizational factors and patients' health beliefs, *Counselling Psychology Quarterly*, 4, 143–55.

Nuckolls K B, Cassel J and Kaplan B H (1972), Psychosocial assets, life crisis and the prognosis of pregnancy, *American Journal of Epidemiology*, 95, 431–41.

O'Leary A (1985), Self-efficacy and health, *Behavior Research and Therapy*, 23, 437–51.

O'Leary A (1990), Stress, emotion and human immune function, *Psychological Bulletin*, 108, 363–82.

O'Reilly P (1988), Methodological issues in social support and social network research, *Social Science and Medicine*, 26, 8, 863–73.

Oakley A (1988), Is social support good for the health of mothers and babies?, *Journal of Infant and Reproductive Psychology*, 6, 3–21.

Oakley A, Rajan L and Grant A (1990), Social support and pregnancy outcome, *British Journal of Obstetrics and Gynaecology*, 97, 155–62.

OPCS: Office of Population Censuses and Surveys (1978), *Occupational Mortality Decenniel Supplement for 1970–72*, London: OPCS.

OPCS: Office of Population Censuses and Surveys (1990), *Standard Occupational Classification*, London: HMSO.

OPCS: Office of Population Censuses and Surveys (1991a), *Mortality Statistics: Cause 1990*, London: HMSO.

OPCS: Office of Population Censuses and Surveys (1991b), *General Household Survey 1989*, London: HMSO.

OPCS: Office of Population Censuses and Surveys (1991c), General Household Survey: cigarette smoking 1972 to 1990, *OPCS Monitor*, SS 91/3, 26 November.

Orth-Gomér K and Undén A-L (1987), The measurement of social support in population surveys, *Social Science and Medicine*, 24, 1, 83–94.

Otis J, Godin G and Lambert J (in press), AIDS prevention: intentions of high school students to use condoms, *Advances in Health Education*.

Parkes C M (1970), The first year of bereavement. A longitudinal study of the reaction of London widows to the death of their husbands, *Psychiatry*, 33, 444–67.

Paykel E S (1978), Contribution of life events to causation of psychiatric illness, *Psychological Medicine*, 8, 245–53.

Paykel E S (1983), Methodological aspects of life events research, *Journal of Psychosomatic Research*, 27, 341–52.

Paykel E S, Prusoff B A and Uhlenhuth E H (1971), Scaling of life events, *Archives of General Psychiatry*, 25, 340–7.

Pearlin L I, Lieberman M A, Menaghan E G and Mullan J P (1981), The stress process, *Journal of Health and Social Behavior*, 22, 337–56.

Pearlin L I and Schooler C (1978), The structure of coping, *Journal of Health and Social Behaviour*, 22, 337–56.

Pendleton D (1983), Doctor–patient communication: a review. In D Pendleton and H Hasler (Eds.), *Doctor–Patient Communication*, London: Academic Press.

Pendleton D and Hasler H (Eds.) (1983), *Doctor–Patient Communication*, London: Academic Press.

Penrose R J J (1972), Life events before subarachnoid haemorrhage, *Journal of Psychosomatic Research*, 16, 329–33.

Peterson C (1988), Explanatory style as a risk factor for illness, *Cognitive Therapy and Research*, 12, 119–32.

Peterson C and Seligman M E P (1986), Content analysis of verbatim explanations: the CAVE technique for assessing explanatory style. Unpublished manuscript, University of Pennsylvania.

Peterson C and Seligman M E P (1987), Explanatory style and illness, *Journal of Personality*, 55, 237–65.

Peterson C, Seligman M E P and Vaillant G E (1988), Pessimistic explanatory style is a risk factor for physical illness: a twenty-five year longitudinal study, *Journal of Personality and Social Psychology*, 55, 23–7.

Peterson C, Semmel A, von Baeyer C, Abramson L Y, Metalsky G I and Seligman M E P (1982), The Attributional Style Questionnaire, *Cognitive Therapy and Research*, 6, 287–300.

Peto R, Lopez A D, Boreham J, Thun M and Heath C (1992), Mortality from tobacco in developed countries: indirect estimation from national vital statistics, *Lancet*, 339, 1268–78.

Pettingale K, Morris T, Greer S and Haybittle J (1985), Mental attitudes to cancer: an additional prognostic factor, *Lancet*, i, 750.

Pocock S J, Shaper A G, Cook D G, Phillips A N and Walker M (1987), Social class differences in ischaemic heart disease in British men, *Lancet*, 25 July, 197–201.

Pohl J M and Fuller S S (1980), Perceived choice, social interaction and dimensions of morale of residents in a home for the aged, *Research in Nursing and Health*, 3, 49–54.

Quine L and Pahl J (1991), Stress and coping in mothers caring for a child with severe learning difficulties: a test of Lazarus' transactional model of coping, *Journal of Community and Applied Social Psychology*, 1, 57–70.

Rabkin J G and Streuning E L (1976), Life events, stress and illness, *Science*, 194, 1013–20.

Ragland D R, Winkleby M A, Schwalbe J, Holman B L, Morse L, Syme S L and Fisher J M (1987), Prevalence of hypertension in bus drivers, *International Journal of Epidemiology*, 16, 208–13.

Rahe R H, McKean J D and Arthur R J (1967), A longitudinal study of life change and illness patterns, *Journal of Psychosomatic Research*, 10, 355–66.

Rahe R H, Meyer E, Smith M, Kjaer S and Holmes T H (1964), Social stress and illness onset, *Journal of Psychosomatic Research*, 8, 35–44.

Roberts R E, Kaplan G A and Camacho T C (1990), Psychological distress and mortality: evidence from the Alemada County Study, *Social Science and Medicine*, 31, 5, 527–36.

Rodin J (1986), Aging and health: effects of the sense of control, *Science*, 233, 1271–6.

Rodin J and Langer E J (1977), Long-term effects of a control-relevant intervention with the institutionalized aged, *Journal of Personality and Social Psychology*, 35, 897–902.

Rolide P, Lewinsohn P M, Tilson M and Seeley J R (1990), Dimensionality of coping and its relation to depression, *Journal of Personality and Social Psychology*, 58, 499–511.

Ronis D L and Harel Y (1989), Health beliefs and breast examination behaviors: analyses of linear structural relations, *Psychology and Health*, 3, 259–85.

Rorsman B, Hagnell O and Lanke J (1982a), Mortality in the Lundby

Study: natural death in different forms of mental disorder in a total population investigated during a 25-year period, *Neuropsychobiology*, 8, 188–97.

Rorsman B, Hagnell O and Lanke J (1982b), Violent death and mental disorder in the Lundby Study: accidents and suicides in a total population during a 25-year period, *Neuropsychobiology*, 8, 233–40.

Rosenman R H (1978), The interview method of assessment of the coronary-prone behavior pattern. In T M Dembroski, S Weiss, J Shields, S G Haynes and M Feinleib (Eds.), *Coronary-Prone Behavior*, 55–69, New York: Springer-Verlag.

Rosenman R H, Brand R J, Jenkins C D, Friedman M, Straus R and Wurm M (1975), Coronary heart disease in the Western Collaborative Group Study: Final follow-up experience of 8½ years, *Journal of the American Medical Association*, 233, 872–7.

Rosenstock I M (1974), Historical origins of the Health Belief Model, *Health Education Monographs*, 2, 328.

Rosentiel A K and Keefe F J (1983), The use of coping strategies in chronic low back pain patients: relationship to patient characteristics and current adjustment, *Pain*, 17, 33–44.

Rotter J B (1966), Generalized expectancies for internal versus external control of reinforcement, *Psychological Monographs*, 80 (1, Whole No. 609).

Royal College of Physicians (1992), *Smoking and the Young*, London: Royal College of Physicians.

Rutter D R and Maguire P (1976), Training medical students to communicate: the development and evaluation of an interviewing model and training procedure. In A E Bennett (Ed.), *Communication Between Doctors and Patients*, 47–74, London: Oxford University Press.

Sarason I G and Spielberger C D (1979), *Stress and Anxiety*, Vol. 6, New York: Hemisphere.

Schaefer C, Coyne J C and Lazarus R S (1981), The health-related functions of social support, *Journal of Behavioral Medicine*, 4, 4, 381–406.

Scheier M F and Carver C S (1985), Optimism, coping and health: assessment and implications of generalized outcome expectancies, *Health Psychology*, 4, 219–47.

Scheier M F and Carver C S (1987), Dispositional optimism and psychological well-being: the influence of generalized outcome expectancies on health, *Journal of Personality*, 55, 169–210.

Scheier M F and Carver C S (1990), What really predicts electoral defeat?, *Psychological Inquiry*, 1, 70–3.

Schifter D B and Ajzen I (1985), Intention, perceived control, and weight loss: an application of the theory of planned behavior, *Journal of Personality and Social Psychology*, 49, 843–51.

Schradle S B and Dougher M J (1985), Social support as a mediator of stress: theoretical and empirical issues, *Clinical Psychology Review*, 5, 641–61.

Schulz R (1976), Effects of control and predictability on the physical and psychological well-being of the institutionalized aged, *Journal of Personality and Social Psychology*, 33, 563–73.

Segall A and Roberts L W (1980), A comparative analysis of physician estimates and levels of medical knowledge among patients, *Sociology of Health and Illness*, 2, 317–34.

Seligman M E P (1975), *Helplessness: On Depression, Development, and Death*, San Francisco: Freeman.

Seligman M E P and Maier S F (1967), Failure to escape traumatic shock, *Journal of Experimental Psychology*, 74, 1–9.

Selye H (1956), *The Stress of Life*, New York: McGraw-Hill.

Shapiro J (1983), Family reactions and coping strategies in response to the physically ill or handicapped child: a review, *Social Science and Medicine*, 17, 14, 913–31.

Sheppard B H, Hartwick J and Warshaw P R (1988), The theory of reasoned action: a meta-analysis of past research with recommendations for modifications and future research, *Journal of Consumer Research*, 15, 325–43.

Sherrod D R (1974), Crowding, perceived control, and behavioral aftereffects, *Journal of Applied Social Psychology*, 4, 171–86.

Shrout P E (1981), Scaling of stressful life events. In B S Dohrenwend and B P Dohrenwend (Eds.), *Stressful Life Events and their Contexts*, 29–47, New York: Prodist.

Simonton D K (1990), Some optimistic thoughts on the pessimistic-rumination thesis, *Psychological Inquiry*, 1, 73–5.

Singer E, Garfunkel R, Cohen S M and Grole L (1976), Mortality and mental health: evidence from the Midtown Manhattan Restudy, *Social Science and Medicine*, 10, 517–25.

Smith G D, Bartley M and Blane D (1990), The Black Report on socioeconomic inequalities in health 10 years on, *British Medical Journal*, 301, 373–7.

Somervell P D, Kaplan B H, Heiss G, Tyroler H A, Kleinbaum D G and Obrist P A (1989), Psychologic distress as a predictor of mortality, *American Journal of Epidemiology*, 130, 1013–23.

Steptoe A (1989), The significance of personal control in health and disease. In A Steptoe and A Appels (Eds.), *Stress, Personal Control and Health*, 309–18, Chichester: Wiley.

Stern J (1983), Social mobility and the interpretation of social class mortality differentials, *Journal of Social Policy*, 12, 27–49.

Strickland B R (1978), Internal–external expectancies and health-related behaviors, *Journal of Consulting and Clinical Psychology*, 46, 1192–211.

Suls J and Fletcher B (1985), The relative efficacy of avoidant and non-avoidant coping strategies: a meta-analysis, *Health Psychology*, 4, 249–88.

Symonds C P (1947), Use and abuse of the term flying stress. In *Air Ministry, Psychological Disorders in Flying Personnel of the Royal Air Force, Investigated during the War 1939–45*, London: HMSO.

Tennant C (1983), Life events and psychological morbidity: the evidence from prospective studies, *Psychological Medicine*, 13, 483–6.

Tennant C (1985), Stress and schizophrenia: a review, *Integrative Psychiatry*, 3, 248–61.

Tennant C (1987), Stress and coronary heart disease, *Australian and New Zealand Journal of Psychiatry*, 21, 276–82.

Tennant C and Andrews G (1978), The pathogenic quality of life event stress in neurotic impairment, *Archives of General Psychiatry*, 35, 859–63.

Tesser A and Shaffer D R (1990), Attitudes and attitude change, *Annual Review of Psychology*, 41, 479–523.

Tetlock P E (1990), Some pessimistic ruminations on disentangling causal processes in presidential elections, *Psychological Inquiry*, 1, 75–6.

Theorell T, Lind E and Floderus B (1975), The relationship of disturbing life changes and emotions to the early development of myocardial infarction and other serious illnesses, *Journal of Epidemiology*, 4, 281–93.

Theorell T and Rahe R H (1971), Psychological factors and myocardial infarction – 1. An inpatient study in Sweden, *Journal of Psychosomatic Research*, 15, 73–88.

Thoits P A (1982), Conceptual, methodological, and theoretical problems in studying social support as a buffer against life stress, *Journal of Health and Social Behavior*, 23, 145–59.

Thoits P A (1985), Social support processes and psychological well-being: theoretical possibilities. In I G Sarason and B Sarason (Eds.), *Social Support: Theory, Research and Applications*, The Hague: Martinus Nijhoff.

Tolman R, Kiff J, Reed S E and Craig W (1980), Predicting experimental colds in volunteers from different measures of recent life stress, *Journal of Psychosomatic Research*, 24, 155–63.

Tsuang M T and Simpson J C (1985), Mortality studies in psychiatry: should they stop or proceed?, *Archives of General Psychiatry*, 42, 98–102.

Vitaliano P P, Russo J, Carr J E, Maiuro R D and Becker J (1985), The ways of coping checklist. Revision and psychometric properties, *Multivariate Behavioural Research*, 20, 3–26.

Wallston B S and Wallston K A (1978), Locus of control and health: a review of the literature, *Health Education Monographs*, 6, 107–17.

Wallston K A (1989), Assessment of control in health-care settings. In A Steptoe and A Appels (Eds.), *Stress, Personal Control and Health*, 85–105, Chichester: Wiley.

Wallston K A, Wallston B S and De Vellis R (1978), Development of the multidimensional health locus of control (MHLC) scales, *Health Education Monographs*, 6, 160–70.

Wallston K A, Wallston B S, Smith M S and Dobbins C J (1987), Perceived control and health, *Current Psychology Research and Reviews*, 6, 5–25.

Weiner B (1985), An attribution theory of achievement motivation and emotion, *Psychological Review*, 92, 548–73.

Weiner B (1986), *An Attributional Theory of Motivation and Emotion*, New York: Springer-Verlag.

Weiner B (1992), *Human Motivation: Metaphors, Theories, and Research*, London: Sage.

Weinstein N D (1980), Unrealistic optimism about future life events, *Journal of Personality and Social Psychology*, 39, 806–20.

Weinstein N D (1982), Unrealistic optimism about susceptibility to health problems, *Journal of Behavioral Medicine*, 5, 441–60.

Weiss R S (1974), The provisions of social relationships. In Z Rubin (Ed.), *Doing Unto Others*, Englewood Cliffs, NJ: Prentice-Hall, 17–26.

Weissman M M, Myers J K, Thompson W K and Belanger A (1986), Depressive symptoms as a risk factor for mortality and for major depression. In L Erlenmeyer-Kimling and N Miller (Eds.), *Life-Span Research and Prediction of Psychopathology*, Potomac, MD: Erlbaum.

Weitz J (1970), Psychological research needs on the problems of human stress. In J E McGrath (Ed.), *Social and Psychological Factors in Stress*, New York: Holt, Rinehart and Winston.

Whitehead M (1987), *The Health Divide: Inequalities in Health in the 1980's*, London: Health Education Council.

WHO: World Health Organization (1987), *World Health Statistics Annual*, Geneva: WHO.

Wicker A W (1969), Attitudes versus actions: the relationship of verbal and overt behavioral responses to attitude objects, *Journal of Social Issues*, 25, 41–78.

Wilkinson R G (1986), Socio-economic differences in mortality:

interpreting the data on their size and trend. In R G Wilkinson (Ed.), *Class and Health*, London: Tavistock, 1–21.

Winkleby M A, Ragland D R and Syme S L (1988), Self-reported stressors and hypertension: evidence of an inverse relationship, *American Journal of Epidemiology*, 27, 124–34.

Zilber N, Schufman N and Lerner Y (1989), Mortality among psychiatric patients in the groups at risk, *Acta Psychiatrica Scandinavica*, 79, 248–53.

Zullow H M and Seligman M E P (1990), Pessimistic rumination predicts defeat of presidential candidates 1900–1984, *Psychological Inquiry*, 1, 52–61.

Chapter 2

Pregnancy Outcome

This year, almost 700,000 children will be born in England and Wales. The huge majority, of course, will thrive, but some 6,000 will die before their first birthday and some 45,000 will weigh less than 2,500 g at birth, placing them at risk. Many of the pregnancies will have complications, and many of the mothers will be dissatisfied with the services they receive. The purpose of this chapter is to identify the main social inputs that affect those outcomes and to trace the social psychological mechanisms that provide the links.

There are four sections. The first presents the published data on pregnancy outcome, and three outcomes are highlighted: early childhood mortality and low birthweight; complications of pregnancy; and satisfaction with maternity care. The second section examines psychosocial risk factors for poor outcome and develops a model in which we draw out the pathways by which we believe the risk factors mediate inputs and outcomes. The principal risk factors we discuss are social factors, including negative life-events and social support; emotional factors, including distress, anxiety, self-esteem and depression; cognitive factors, including knowledge, beliefs and attitudes to pregnancy; coping resources and strategies; and behavioural factors, including take-up of services, smoking, drinking, diet and work. The third section of the chapter reports our own programme of research; and the concluding section discusses the implications of our findings for theory, policy, and practice.

Indices of pregnancy outcome

Early childhood mortality and low birthweight

In the mid-nineteenth century more than 15 per cent of children in England and Wales died before their first birthday (Figure 2.1). At the turn of the century the figure was little changed, but then a steep decline began as rudimentary state health care and later the full National Health Service developed. By 1960 the figure was just over 2 per cent, and in 1984 it fell below 1 per cent for the first time. Comparable data for the European Community and the rest of Europe, however, show that Britain's record is poor, especially compared with Scandinavia and most other West European countries. Indeed it is deteriorating for, between 1970–5 and 1985–90, Britain slipped three places out of twenty-four, from tenth to thirteenth.

Infant mortality is an important measure of a nation's health,

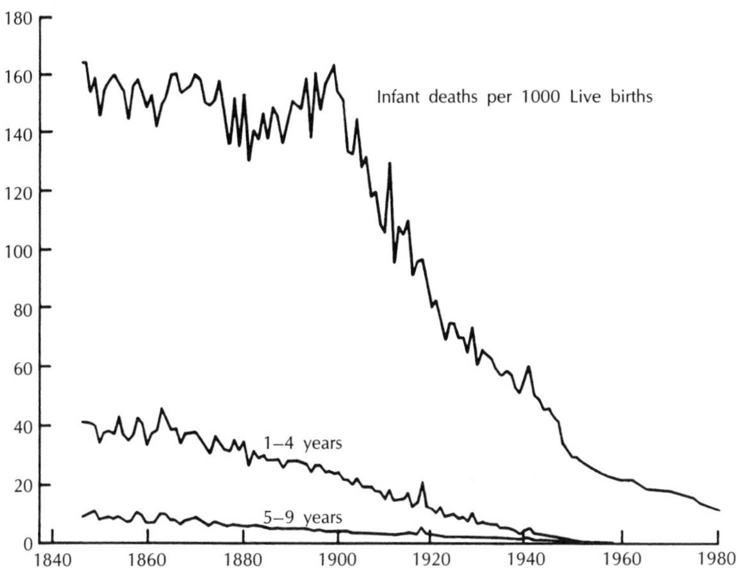

Figure 2.1 Infant and childhood mortality in England and Wales, 1846–1981. Source: Macfarlane and Mugford (1984)

which the World Health Organization has included as one of the twelve indicators in its Global Strategy for Health for All by the Year 2000, as we saw in Chapter 1. Beyond crude overall rates, however, it is useful to break down the figures by the precise age at death, for in that way the possible causes of the secular trends may begin to emerge: stillbirths; neonatal deaths (0–27 days); post-neonatal deaths (28 days–12 months); and infant deaths (under 1 year after live birth). The most noticeable features of the data are the steady decline in the overall rates for stillbirths and neonatal deaths, but the unsteady trend for post-neonatal mortality, where the figures for 1982, 1985 and 1986 all increased over the immediately preceding year (Figure 2.2). The effect of the marked increase in post-neonatal mortality in 1986 was to increase the infant mortality ratio in that year too. For all the indices in 1989 the overall figure was 60 per cent to 65 per cent of the 1980 figure, except for post-neonatal mortality where it was almost 85 per cent. Sudden Infant Death Syndrome accounted for more than half the post-neonatal deaths, with congenital abnormalities the second most frequent cause.

Perhaps the most striking finding to emerge is the significance of social class. It is well established that the greatest risk at birth is to children of mothers who are older or have had several children already (Macfarlane and Mugford, 1984). However, even when age and parity are controlled, mortality rates during the first year are found to be strongly class-related. All the data are based on the father's occupation, and for each of the indices there is a steady gradient from low mortality in Social Class I to high mortality in Social Class V. When the data are expressed as ratios between Class V and Class I, even in 1989 they were considerable – 1.8 : 1 for infant mortality overall (Figure 2.3), 2.1 : 1 for stillbirths, 1.3 : 1 for neonatal mortality and 2.7 : 1 for post-neonatal mortality (Figure 2.4). The figure for post-neonatal mortality is particularly important because the child who dies after the first month of life will normally have been discharged from hospital, and deficiencies in NHS neonatal care are therefore less likely to play a part than domestic social and environmental factors. Consistent with this argument, the *causes* of post-neonatal mortality, unlike the overall *rates*, are distributed evenly across the classes, indicating that children at the bottom of the social scale suffer *general* vulnerability.

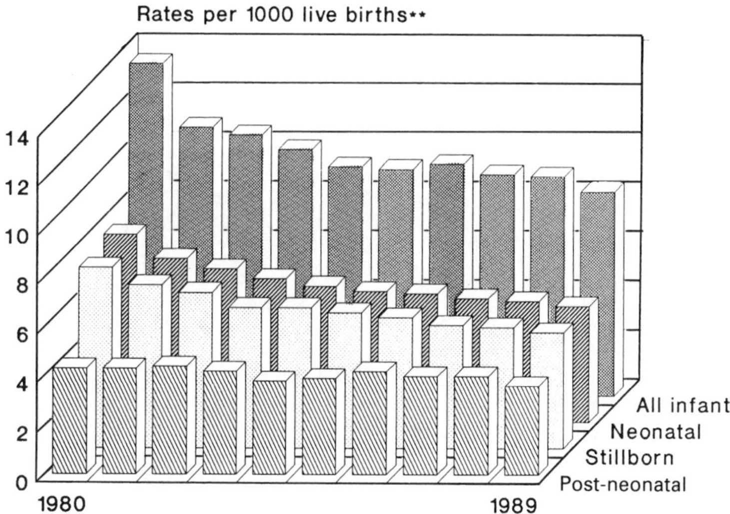

Figure 2.2 Infant mortality in England and Wales*. Source: OPCS Series DH3. (*Illegitimate births are included. **Per 1,000 total births for stillborn.)

Middle-class circumstances offer overall, non-specific protection.

The other principal 'hard' index of pregnancy outcome is low birthweight, which is now normally defined as 2,499 g or less. A reduction in the number of low-weight births is another of the WHO's global indicators for the year 2000, and international comparisons produce a similar pattern to the figures for infant mortality. Indeed, the two are closely related, in part, of course, because mortality among low birthweight babies is high. Once more there is a sharp difference between the top and bottom of the social scale in England and Wales, with ratios for Class V to Class I of 1.6 : 1, even in 1989. Useful reviews of both population-based and hospital-based analyses are to be found in Peters *et al.* (1983), Ounsted, Moar and Scott (1985), Carr-Hill (1987) and Pickering (1987a, 1987b).

The most telling data, however, are for low-birthweight children who die early in childhood. For both perinatal and infant mortality among low-birthweight children, there has been a sharp

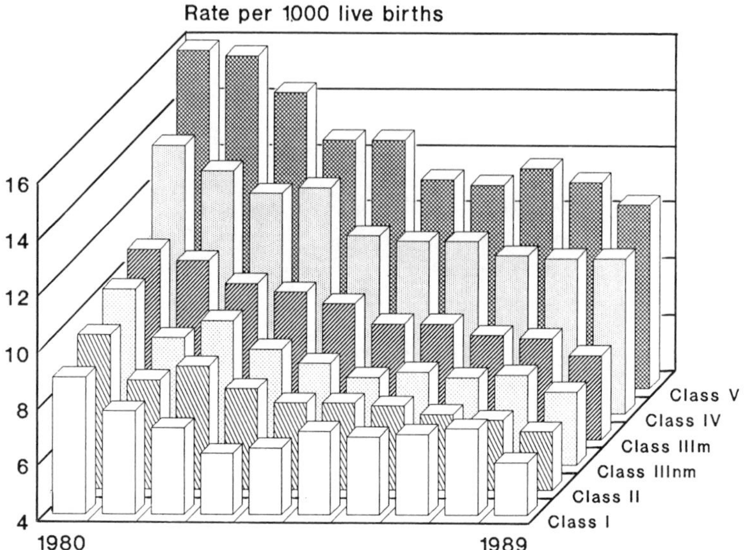

Figure 2.3 Infant mortality by social class. Source: OPCS Series DH3

decline in the 1980s in England and Wales, so that improvements in neonatal care are today keeping alive some 30 per cent or 40 per cent of babies who, as recently as 1980, would have died. Even so, more than two-thirds of those who die are lost within seven days of birth, the early neonatal period. What also emerges is that, just as for mortality among babies overall, deaths among low-birthweight babies are again class-related, though the ratios this time are less marked and have shown greater signs of improvement with the years (Figure 2.5). Low-birthweight children who survive have high rates of medical and developmental problems (see the recent work of, for example, Lloyd, 1984; Alberman, Benson and Kani, 1985; Nelson and Ellenberg, 1986; Stanley and English, 1986; Marlow, D'Souza and Chiswick, 1987; Skeoch *et al.*, 1987) – and increased survival is likely to mean more infant morbidity overall – but whether those rates too are class-related is not known.

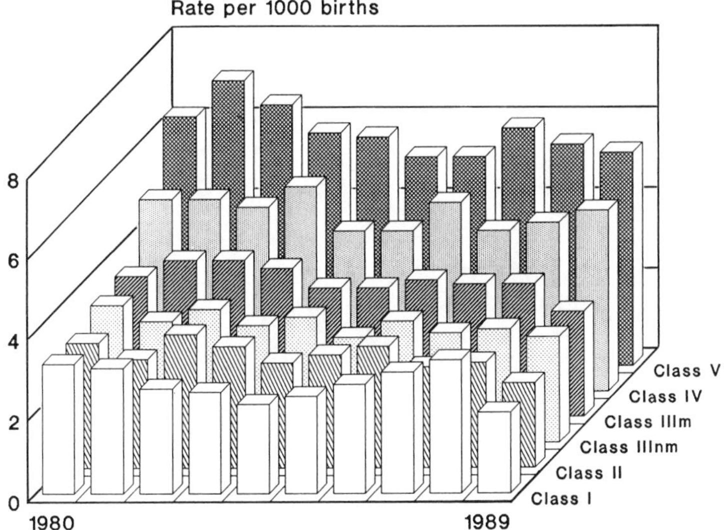

Figure 2.4 Post-neonatal mortality by social class. Source: OPCS Series DH3

Complications of pregnancy

Recent national figures for complications of pregnancy, labour and delivery are more difficult to find. The Hospital In-Patient Enquiry (HIPE), the most useful source, has now been discontinued, and the 1982–5 HIPE maternity tables (OPCS, 1988) therefore provide the most recent figures available. The most important measure is the estimated total maternity discharges (of delivered women only) by complications (Figure 2.6). A very wide range of complications is included: those related mainly to pregnancy such as antepartum haemorrhage, hypertension and early or threatened labour; those that indicate the need for greater care in pregnancy, labour and delivery, such as multiple gestation, malpresentation of the foetus or suspected fetal abnormality; complications occurring mainly in the course of labour, such as long labour or postpartum haemorrhage; and complications of the puerperium, such as puerperal infection or obstetrical pulmonary embolism.

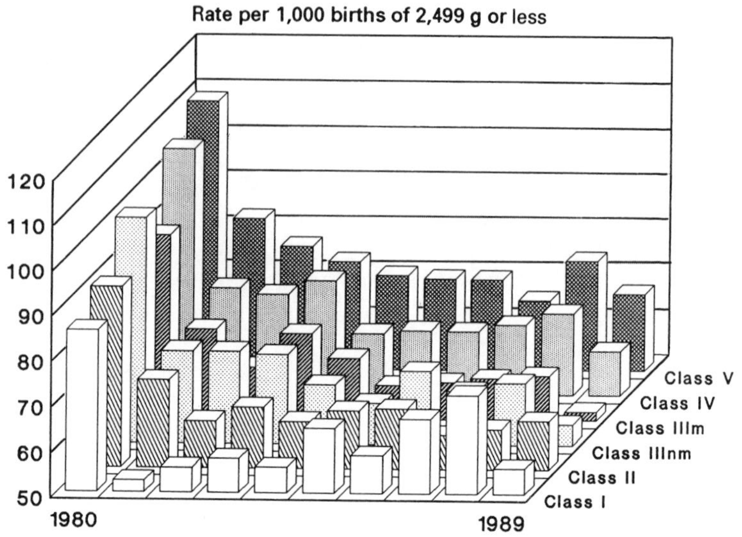

Figure 2.5 Infant mortality by low birthweight. Source: OPCS Series DH3 and Monitors

Of 605,120 deliveries in 1985, only 37.9 per cent were considered uncomplicated. This compares with 45 per cent in 1975 and 45 per cent in 1980, so the trend is towards more complications being reported. Estimated *total* complications for 1984 were 641,780. Women can have more than one complication, so this figure is based on the number of complications mentioned rather than on the number of women. Thus, for example, hypertension constituted 8.3 per cent of the total complications, early or threatened labour 4 per cent, long labour 5.7 per cent and obstetrical trauma 12.3 per cent. Women experiencing complications are more likely to give birth to a baby with complications than women experiencing a problem-free pregnancy – 22 per cent in 1985, for example, against 7 per cent (OPCS, 1988, Series MB4, No 28, Table 7.5). The national figures are not broken down by social class, but there are indications from the literature that some pregnancy complications *are* related to it (for example, Butler, 1969; Fedrick and

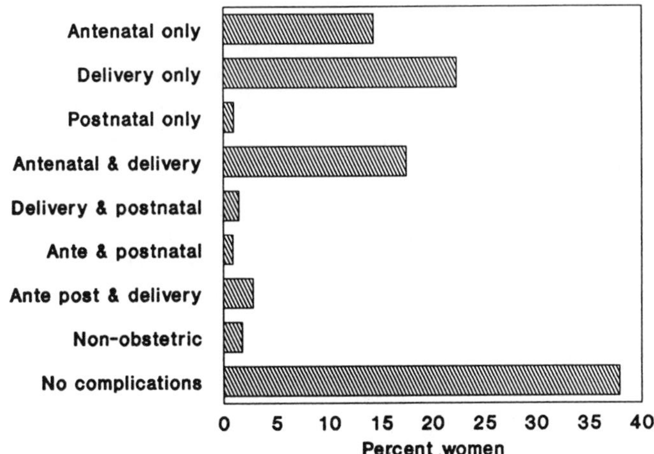

Figure 2.6 Pregnancy complications: England (1985). Data are for delivered women only. Source: OPCS Series MB4

Anderson, 1976; Elbourne, Pritchard and Daurncey, 1986; Sanjose, Ramon and Beral, 1991).

Satisfaction with maternity care

From early childhood mortality and low birthweight, and pregnancy complications, we turn now to 'soft' outcomes of pregnancy, which are often ignored: women's experience and satisfaction with maternity care, their assessment of the quality of their birth experience, and medical communications during and after pregnancy. In 1981 the Secretaries of State for Social Services and for Wales set up the Maternity Services Advisory Committee to advise on matters relating to maternity and neonatal services. In their First Report (Maternity Services Advisory Committee, 1982), the Committee voiced their concern about 'the number of consumer complaints about the so-called impersonal nature of care in hospitals where maternity services are now concentrated'. It recommended that District Health

Authorities should set up a Maternity Services Liaison Committee which would monitor consumers' views on the quality of care and aim to raise levels of satisfaction among users. OPCS was requested to develop a survey manual that could be used by DHAs wishing to measure consumers' views of local maternity services, and the result was *Women's Experience of Maternity Care – A Postal Survey Manual* (HMSO, 1989). Data based on a representative national sample of DHAs showed that 59 per cent of mothers were very satisfied, 40 per cent were satisfied in some ways but not in others, and only 1 per cent were very dissatisfied. The aspect of care that generated both the most favourable and the most unfavourable comments was 'aspects of personal relations, communications and/or amount of time given by the staff' (Figure 2.7).

Other studies have produced similar findings (Cartwright, 1979; Graham and McKee, 1979; Reid and McIlwaine, 1980; O'Brien and Smith, 1981; Green, Coupland and Kitzinger, 1990). Graham and McKee (1979), for example, found that 90 per cent of mothers in a sample of 200 thought that antenatal care was important, but 34 per cent felt they did not have the opportunity

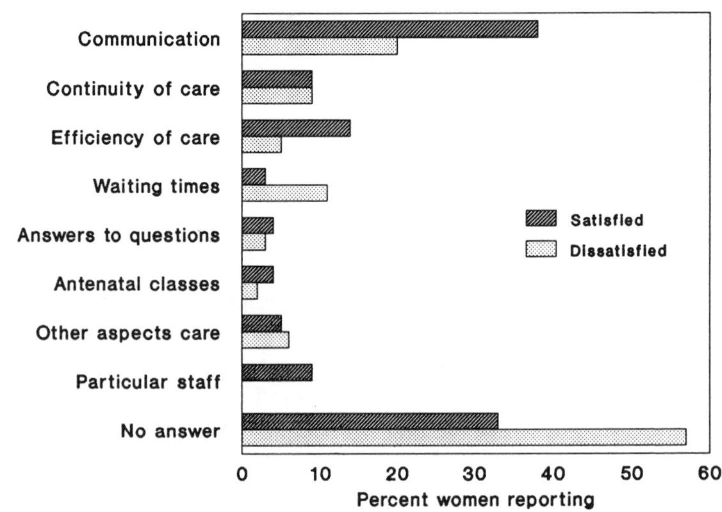

Figure 2.7 Satisfaction with antenatal care. Source: OPCS (1989)

to ask questions, 52 per cent said they did not enjoy their visits, and 80 per cent said they had not learned anything from their clinic check-ups. Green, Coupland and Kitzinger (1990) found that overall satisfaction was related to whether women felt they had received the 'right' amount of information, and whether they expected the birth to be painful. Cartwright (1979) found that working-class mothers wanted information about their pregnancy as much as middle-class mothers, but that they were less successful at obtaining it. The number of topics about which mothers would have liked more information rose from 3.3 in Social Class I to 5.5 in Social Class V. In each of the studies, it is interesting to note that *medical communications* have often been the major source of dissatisfaction, as in many other studies of health care provision (Ley, 1988).

The OPCS study did not analyze or comment on social class differences in satisfaction, but other researchers, such as Hubert (1974), Cartwright (1979) and Nelson (1983), have found marked effects. Nelson (1983), for example, in an important American study, found that working-class women were likely to have negative feelings about pregnancy, while middle-class women felt that pregnancy, labour, delivery and the baby were interrelated pleasures. Working-class women were also more apprehensive about labour and delivery and the discomfort they might feel, and were more likely to favour interventions during birth – medication during labour and delivery, artificial rupture of membranes, delivery room births and fetal monitoring – which they were then more likely to receive. The differences between the classes in attitudes and experience led in turn to differences in satisfaction: middle-class women were more likely to complain about personality conflicts with staff, mismanagement of labour and the fact that medication was offered too frequently, while working-class women complained about the lack of information offered during labour and delivery, and about the pain and discomfort. Nelson concluded that there are two distinct models of childbirth which have their roots in the different life experiences of middle- and working-class women. For working-class women, a painless, technological birth process will produce satisfaction, while middle-class women want participation and personal control over labour with as little medical intervention as possible.

Social inputs and mediators: psychosocial risk factors and a theoretical model

It is clear from the preceding review that one of the most important social inputs affecting pregnancy outcome is social class. What emerges is a downward trend towards adverse pregnancy outcomes through the social classes, a pattern that has been reported many times throughout the health literature on children and adults alike, as we saw in Chapter 1. Our concern now is to determine *how* social class has its effects upon outcome. First we examine in detail the psychosocial risk factors known to be associated with poor pregnancy outcome, and then we develop a theoretical model, in which the risk factors are seen as mediators between inputs and outcomes.

Psychosocial risk factors

Life-events and social support

In a well-known study by Brown and Harris (1978), working-class women with children at home were found to suffer almost three times as many 'severe household events' as middle-class women – serious illness or injury, substantial reduction in income, marital breakdown, and so on. Newton *et al.* (1979) went on to show that a high frequency of life-events during pregnancy was associated with pre-term births, and Newton and Hunt (1984), in a prospective study, reported that working-class women had significantly more life-events during their pregnancies than middle-class women, and that life-events were associated with low birthweight. An even better predictor of low birthweight was smoking during pregnancy, which the authors suggested was a mediator of stress, as Graham (1976, 1984) too has argued. Thus, working-class women, especially with children at home, were likely to suffer more frequent life-events than were middle-class women, and life-events were associated with pre-term and low-birthweight outcomes, both directly in their own right and indirectly through smoking. Similar findings have been reported many times (see the reviews by Oakley, MacFarlane and Chalmers, 1982; Oakley, 1985; Levin and DeFrank, 1988; Pagel *et al.*, 1990).

What the literature also suggests, however, is that threatening life-events can to some extent be counteracted or 'buffered' if the woman has social support, in the way that Henderson has argued more generally in his theoretical work on social networks and social support (Henderson, Byrne and Duncan-Jones, 1981). A study of social support intervention in pregnancy involving 507 women (Oakley and Rajan, 1991) found that extra social support in pregnancy was associated with a statistically significant improvement in some health outcomes, such as hospital admission in pregnancy, use of neonatal intensive care by babies, health service use by mothers and babies, and psychological parameters of well-being, especially anxiety. Oakley and Rajan found that working-class women are more isolated in terms of friends than middle-class women, and receive less male domestic support. Nuckolls, Cassel and Kaplan (1972), in a study of army wives, examined the relationship of stressful life-events and 'psycho-social assets' (such as social support and self-esteem) to pregnancy complications. Though neither was related to increased risk when examined alone, high stress (life-events) was associated with complications of both pregnancy and delivery when social supports were absent. When stress and social support were both split at the median in a subsequent re-analysis by Cobb (1976), 91 per cent of women with high stress but low social support were found to have complications, against only 33 per cent with high stress and high social support, a difference which was highly significant statistically. Cobb's paper was the 1976 Presidential Address to the American Psychosomatic Society, and it provides a useful review of the literature on social support as a buffer, in pregnancy and many other health-related areas. Other reviews of the conceptual and theoretical issues are to be found in Dean and Lin (1977), Antonovsky (1979), Thoits (1982), Fox (1988) and O'Reilly (1988).

Many other studies have been reported – some using description, others intervention – and some of the most interesting recent research has concentrated on providing immediate support during the confinement and the birth itself. Simply having another woman present at the birth, it has been argued, leads to shorter labour, fewer complications during labour and delivery, fewer admissions to neonatal intensive care and an increase in mother–infant interaction in the first minutes after the birth (Sosa *et al.*, 1980; Klaus *et al.*, 1986; Hofmeyer *et al.*, 1991). Social support throughout the pregnancy is claimed to reduce the incidence of low birthweight and pregnancy complications (see the review by Oakley, 1985). Support immediately after the birth, especially if given by professionally trained staff, may also help to reduce the mother's anxiety during the first year of the child's life (Barnett and Parker, 1985; Parker and Barnett, 1987).

Emotional factors: maternal distress, anxiety, self-esteem and depression

It is well established that emotional factors have a significant effect on a variety of pregnancy outcomes from low birthweight to complications of pregnancy and satisfaction with the birth experience (for example, Oakley *et al.*, 1982; Levin and DeFrank, 1988), and in the last decade progress has been made in uncovering the physiological mechanisms by which they operate on labour, delivery, and so on. Lederman *et al.* (1978, 1979), for example, found that measurements of state anxiety during labour correlated significantly with uterine contractions and length of labour. Anxiety was also related, though, to attitudes towards the pregnancy, and it is psychological processes on which much of the most recent literature has concentrated. Wolkind and Zajicek (1981), for example, in their longitudinal research on pregnancy and mothering in the East End of London, found that the average weight of children born to mothers with a diagnosed psychiatric condition was significantly lower than for children with psychiatrically healthy mothers. The disturbed mothers were on average younger, attended antenatal classes less frequently and smoked more – and it was smoking that predicted low birthweight best of all. According to Brown and Harris (1978), as we have seen, the most likely women to suffer depression are working-class women at home with small children and significant numbers of severe life-events – and now, according to Wolkind and Zajicek (1981), psychiatric illness is associated with low birthweight. The evidence thus begins to suggest a complex pattern of relationships between social class and outcome, with psychosocial risk factors acting as mediators.

In another important study, Norbeck and Tilden (1983) investigated the effects upon pregnancy outcome of life stress, social support, and 'emotional disequilibrium', a construct made up of state anxiety, depression and low self-esteem. Life stress, social support and emotional disequilibrium were found to be interrelated, but each had separate effects, in that life stress predicted gestational difficulties, while emotional disequilibrium was associated with complications in the infant's health. When life stress and social support were examined together – that is, when stress was present but social support was absent – complications were noted in a whole range of outcomes, including gestation, labour and delivery, and the infant's condition. The findings were thus consistent with the stress-buffering effect of social support noted earlier.

Other studies have explored a variety of related concepts – including trait and state anxiety (Beck *et al.*, 1980; Lunenfield *et al.*, 1984; Newton and Hunt, 1984), psychodynamic defences (McDonald, 1968) and maternal distress (Blomberg, 1980). Some writers argue that psychological and life stress variables do not function independently but work in synergy (Obayuwana, Carter and Barnett, 1984; Molfese *et al.*, 1987; Pagel *et al.*, 1990). A useful review of the entire area is to be found in Oakley *et al.* (1982). 'One might say', Oakley concludes, that working-class women are 'with good reason, more anxious and doubtful of any possibility of controlling what happens to them' (Oakley *et al.*, 1982, p. 17). One might also speculate that reducing anxiety and depression is precisely the role played by social support in buffering the effects of life-events (see, for example, O'Hara, 1986).

Cognitive factors

Knowledge. Research on knowledge as a mediator of health behaviours and outcomes has adopted two main approaches, the first of which is descriptive. The most influential model has been that of Ley (Ley and Spelman, 1967; Ley, 1982), whose main concern has been to describe the relationships between cognitive variables and patients' satisfaction, particularly their satisfaction with medical communications. The most important predictors, the model argues, are comprehension and memory, and satisfaction will in turn lead to compliance. In the absence of knowledge, comprehension and memory will be low, and so, in turn, will satisfaction and compliance.

In the case of pregnancy, almost all the research has been of the second type, which consists of intervention studies. The main interest has been in testing whether providing knowledge through antenatal classes, for example, leads to more appropriate behaviours and more positive outcomes. Reviews of the effects of classes on behaviour are to be found in Westbrook (1979), Beck *et al.* (1980) and Nelson (1982), and reviews of research on the links between classes and outcome are to be found in Enkin (1982), Bakketeig, Hoffman and Oakley (1984) and Rutter, Quine and Hayward (1988). In neither area is the evidence entirely consistent, but the overall trend is towards positive relationships.

Beliefs. Much the most important stimulus to research on health beliefs has been the Health Belief Model of Becker and his colleagues (Janz and Becker, 1984). As we saw in Chapter 1, the model argues that health behaviours – taking up services, reducing smoking, changing diet, and so on, as ways of preventing pregnancy complications – will be predicted by three main variables: how vulnerable the woman perceives herself to be to the complications; how severe or important she believes them to be; and how she weighs the benefits and costs of taking action.

Following a suggestion by Becker (1976), that the translation of health beliefs into action requires a trigger to reinforce the personal relevance of the information, Reading *et al.* (1982) investigated the possible role of ultrasound scanning. Women who were scanned at their first antenatal visit were either given high feedback, in which they were shown the size and shape of the fetus and its movements were pointed out, or they were given no picture and no specific verbal description or comments. At the same visit, all the women were given advice about smoking and drinking. At follow-up, significantly more of those given feedback than those given nothing were found to have followed the advice.

Few other writers have used the Health Belief Model for examining pregnancy, but three studies have used Fishbein and Ajzen's Theory of Reasoned Action (Fishbein and Ajzen, 1975). Manstead, Profitt and Smart (1983) predicted who from a group of mothers-to-be would choose to breastfeed, and who would not; Godin and LePage (1988) used the model to predict the intentions of first-time mothers to smoke cigarettes after childbirth; and Lowe and Frey (1983) used it to predict intentions to use the Lamaze method of childbirth. In each case, the model showed that beliefs played an important role.

Attitudes to pregnancy. Several studies have investigated the effects on pregnancy outcome of women's attitudes towards pregnancy, but the findings are by no means clear (B. Chalmers, 1982). Yang *et al.* (1976), for example, found that pregnant women with many fears concerning childbirth and motherhood were more likely to have longer labours and to require more drugs. 'Negative' attitudes towards pregnancy and motherhood have been found to be related to vomiting during pregnancy (Chertok, 1972), prolonged labour (Kapp, Horstein and Graham, 1963), pain during labour (Nettelbladt, Fagerstom and Uddenberg, 1976; Beck *et al.*, 1980) and high levels of medication (Doering and Entwisle, 1975), toxaemia (Ringrose, 1972) and prematurity (Blau *et al.*, 1963; Grimm, 1967). Moreover, a carefully designed prospective study by Molfese *et al.* (1987) found that attitudes towards pregnancy, together with social support and locus of control, acted as mediators between maternal anxiety, depression and life stress, and measures of infant postnatal status.

Other research has led to rather different conclusions. Zajicek (1981), for example, could find no relationship between attitudes to pregnancy and motherhood and either length of labour or drug dosage. B. Chalmers (1983, 1984), however, found 'positive' attitudes to be predictive of complications. The reason, he argued, was that social support can sometimes lead to denial of anxiety, and that what the woman needs is the opportunity to 'work through' the fear. The important aspect of social support was quality rather than quantity. In one final study, conducted some years earlier, Rosengren (1961) found that many women regarded pregnancy as a physical illness and that they were more likely to be from working-class backgrounds. Moreover, there was a positive relationship between adoption of the sick role and length of labour but, interestingly, the relationship was affected by the obstetrician's attitudes, for labour lasted longer when the doctor and the woman had incongruous views.

As to why attitudes should be important, Grimm (1967) has

argued that they may influence the woman's behaviour during pregnancy – posture, diet, smoking, drinking, how early she visits a doctor for antenatal care, how well she takes care of herself, and so on – all of which, in turn, may affect the outcome of the pregnancy. Such behaviours, he argues, may also be influenced by antenatal classes.

Coping resources and strategies

With coping resources and strategies we reach the nub of psychosocial mediators, for it is in how women cope with their pregnancy that many of the psycho-social mediators are drawn together. As we saw in Chapter 1, coping has been defined as the problem-solving efforts made by an individual when the demands of a given situation tax adaptive resources (Lazarus, Averill and Opton, 1974; Pearlin and Schooler, 1978). The central process is cognitive appraisal, which is a mental process by which people assess whether a demand threatens their well-being (primary appraisal), appraise their resources for meeting the demand, formulate solutions, and select strategies (secondary appraisal). For a number of women, we suggest, lack of *material* resources may result in a reduced choice of coping strategies. Lack of *physical* resources may mean that pre-existing physical or psychological ill-health will impede the process of coping. Lack of *social* resources may mean that fewer people can be called upon to help. Lack of *psychological* and *intellectual* resources may produce cognitive problems that include an inability to respond to difficulties in optimistic, persistent and flexible ways; an explanatory style that focuses on the internal, stable and global factors of negative events; and low self-efficacy. Pregnancy care will be seen as the responsibility of outside professionals, and internal locus of control will be weak. This may lead in turn to the selection and use of ineffectual coping strategies, and the likely result will be a willingness to take potentially dangerous behavioural risks, whether failing to carry out positive measures, such as taking up antenatal services, or continuing to pursue negative behaviours, such as smoking. The central issue is whether such women can be identified and classified.

The answer appears to be that many are from working-class backgrounds of material deprivation. Some of the best-known evidence of a relationship between social class and coping strategies comes from Pill and Stott (1982, 1985), who explored concepts of illness causation and responsibility in working-class women. Those who were less well educated and of lower socioeconomic status were significantly more likely to hold fatalistic views about illness causation and to deny personal responsibility for their health – that is, they were low in internal locus of control (Wallston and Wallston, 1978a, 1978b, 1981). Blaxter has reached similar conclusions (Blaxter and Paterson, 1982; Blaxter, 1985, 1987), and Pill and Stott (1987), in their more recent work on the development of the Salience of Lifestyle Index, have gone on to show that whether or not people perceive their daily decisions about smoking, diet, exercise, and so on as choices that determine future health is also related to educational status. In the case of pregnancy, such views are likely to lead to a willingness to take risks with health and an unwillingness to accept that 'positive' behaviours, such as taking exercise, giving up smoking, reducing alcohol intake and maintaining a good diet, might influence outcome.

Other research has been conducted on the role of antenatal education in reducing stress and increasing coping behaviour, and one especially interesting example comes from a prospective study by Doering, Entwisle and Quinlan (1980), based on Janis's theory of stress and coping (Janis, 1958). Preparation for childbirth, it was found, whether from classes, books, television, or indeed any other source, was associated with a more enjoyable birth, because the prepared women needed less medication and anaesthesia than the others and so were able to retain awareness and control. The husband's support and presence emerged as an important second factor and, together, preparation and support accounted for more than half the variance in the dependent measures.

Behavioural factors

Take-up of services. Although antenatal care and maternity services are free to everyone in Britain, many mothers-to-be register their pregnancies late and fail to attend antenatal classes regularly, while some are not even known to the services until labour itself begins. Failure to take up services can have serious consequences, as Greenberg (1983) was able to show in a powerful analysis of US data. All births in the United States were examined from official statistics for one year, and it emerged that poorly educated black women were almost nine times less likely to register for antenatal care than were well-educated white women. Low birthweight was almost three times as common in the former as the latter, and it was in the poorly educated black group that the strongest association between low birthweight and failure to take up services emerged – almost six times the figure for the well-educated white group. The very people, in other words, whom antenatal care might have benefited most were the ones least likely to receive it. A similar pattern of associations was reported by Lewis (1982) for working-class women in this country.

It is well established that registering the pregnancy late, and subsequently failing to attend antenatal appointments and preparation classes, are associated with descending social class (McKinlay, 1970, 1973; McKinlay and McKinlay, 1979; Scott-Samuel, 1980; Simpson and Walker, 1980; O'Brien and Smith, 1981). Most of the research that has tried to find an explanation, however, has concentrated on the woman, and only recently has attention turned to the characteristics of the care and the possible mismatch between care and consumers (Reid and McIlwaine, 1980; I. Chalmers, 1984; Taylor, 1986). At least part of the problem, the more recent evidence suggests, is the structural organization of the health care system, with its current emphasis on hospital-based services at the expense of general practice and local health centre care (Cavenagh *et al.*, 1984; Robson, Boomla and Savage, 1986; Young, 1987).

Smoking. An excellent summary of research on smoking and pregnancy outcome appeared in the Fourth Report of the Independent Scientific Committee on Smoking and Health (Froggatt, 1988). Smoking during pregnancy has been shown many times to be associated with fetal and neonatal mortality, low birthweight and developmental retardation (US Surgeon General, 1980; UK Royal College of Physicians, 1983; Abel, 1984), and indeed the first evidence appeared as early as 1957 (Simpson, 1957). For mothers who smoke, the increase in perinatal mortality is estimated at 28 per cent, the reduction in birthweight is 150–250 g on average, and the risk of having a low birthweight baby is doubled (see the reviews by Bakketeig *et al.*, 1984; and Simpson and Smith, 1986). Simpson and Smith go so far as to say that smoking is responsible for 20 per cent of all low-weight births in this country. All the reported effects increase with the number of cigarettes smoked but, if the mother changes her behaviour before the end of the fourth month of pregnancy, the risk to the baby is determined by the new pattern of behaviour and not the original one. Recent evidence suggests that so-called 'passive smoking' – exposure to environmental tobacco smoke produced by other people – may also be associated with reduced birthweight (Martin and Bracken, 1986; Rubin *et al.*, 1986).

Although these studies provide evidence that the association is causal and serious, some researchers have claimed that the correlation may be spurious (Yerushalmy, 1971; Oakley, 1989). Oakley, for example, argues that smoking in pregnancy is linked to various aspects of women's maternal and social position. Working-class women experience poorer material conditions and lower social support, which makes negative life-events and chronic long-term difficulties more likely. These in turn lead to stress. Smoking is a coping strategy used in response both to stress and to impoverished material and social conditions.

An important point to emerge from Froggatt (1988), in contrast, is that the effects of smoking during pregnancy appear to operate *independently* of potentially confounding factors, such as social class, parity, the mother's age and height, and the sex of the child – though there are, of course, marked differences in the incidence of smoking by social group. For example, more than twice as many women smoke in Class V as in Class I – 36 per cent against 16 per cent according to OPCS data for 1990 (OPCS, 1991a). Data from the British Perinatal Mortality Survey and the British Births Survey indicate that 41.3 per cent of pregnant women smoked in 1970 against 29.5 per cent in 1958 (Peters *et al.*, 1983), and the equivalent estimate made by Simpson and Smith (1986) for their 1984 data based on the General Household Survey was 29 per cent, ranging from 13 per cent in Class I to 31.5 per cent in Class V. The implication is that most women who smoke continue to do so during pregnancy: pregnancy does not stop them.

Further evidence against non-causal explanations of the

association between smoking and low birthweight come from the results of randomized intervention trials, in which mothers-to-be were encouraged to stop smoking during pregnancy. There have been three. The first, by Donovan (1977), was inconclusive, but produced some indication of an increase in birthweight in comparison with a control group whose mothers continued to smoke. The second, by Sexton and Habel (1984), showed that among singletons 'experimental' babies were born an average of 92 g heavier and 0.6 cm longer than 'control' babies; and the third, by MacArthur, Newton and Knox (1987), produced figures of 68 g and 0.75 cm. Intervention studies offer the best evidence so far of a causal link, but whether the link is a direct physiological one or is mediated through the effects of stress buffering and support, for example, has yet to be determined (Sexton and Habel, 1984).

From one final piece of evidence, produced by the Oxford Family Planning Association Study, it has emerged that even smoking before pregnancy may be important (Howe *et al.*, 1985). Of women who were smoking twenty or more cigarettes a day when they entered the study, which was some time before they hoped to conceive, 11 per cent had still not produced a baby five years after they stopped contraception, against 5 per cent for non-smokers. The effect was independent of social class.

Drinking. The findings for drinking are more complex. It is established that heavy drinking during pregnancy, defined as 80 g or more of alcohol a day, can lead to the Foetal Alcohol Syndrome. Research has also indicated that more moderate levels of intake may be associated with a wide variety of fetal problems such as increased incidence of stillbirths, spontaneous abortion, congenital abnormalities and growth retardation (Waterson and Murray-Lyon, 1990). Some of the findings are inconsistent, but there is general acceptance that moderate alcohol consumption is related to fetal growth retardation (Wright *et al.*, 1983; Barrison, Waterson and Murray-Lyon, 1985). In the early 1980s, the recommendation was that women should avoid alcohol altogether during pregnancy (US Surgeon General, 1981; UK Royal College of Psychiatrists, 1982).

There was a considerable body of evidence. Wright *et al.* (1983), for example, in a prospective study of almost 1,000 women, found that those who were heavy drinkers at the time of conception (100 g or more a week) ran twice the risk of light drinkers (0–50 g) of producing a baby in the lowest 10 per cent for weight. For moderate drinkers (50–100 g), the figure was 1.25: 1. This was significantly increased for women who smoked and were in Social Classes III, IV and V. A prospective study by Russell and Skinner (1988) found that two reported measures of maternal alcohol misuse before pregnancy were associated with adverse pregnancy outcomes. Average ounces of absolute alcohol consumed per day predicted spontaneous abortion and lowered Apgar scores. Indicators of problem drinking predicted problems of uterine growth, lower Apgar scores and low birthweight. A review by Barrison and Wright (1984) cites several studies that suggest that even moderate drinking (50–100 g alcohol per day) may be harmful. A prospective study by Little (1977) found that a daily intake of 2–3 drinks in early pregnancy reduced birthweight by 3 g for each gm of alcohol taken. Grisso *et al.* (1984), however, in a similar prospective study, suggested that women who were regular drinkers before pregnancy produced *heavier* babies – but only frequency of drinking was measured and quantity and type of alcohol went unrecorded. Low birthweight accounted for 7.5–8 per cent of births in light, moderate and heavy drinkers alike.

One of the problems for interpretation – and perhaps one of the reasons for inconsistencies in the literature – is that drinking is often associated with smoking, and the effects are sometimes difficult to disentangle (see the recent research of Little *et al.*, 1986; Rubin *et al.*, 1986; and Sulaiman *et al.*, 1988). For example, the social class distributions for drinking and smoking are opposite – most heavy drinkers are middle-class, most heavy smokers working-class – but the group with the highest proportion of heavy drinkers, 42 per cent, is smokers in Classes I and II (Wright *et al.*, 1983). The risk of producing a baby in the lowest 10 per cent for weight, Wright *et al.* found, was 3.4 times as great for heavy drinkers who were smokers as for women who neither drank nor smoked.

As to the relationship with social class, Brooke *et al.* (1989) found that women who come from materially deprived situations or who smoke are more likely to produce children with lower birthweight. These factors may interact and increase the risk, as smoking and drinking do (Wright *et al.*, 1983). Studies in the United States conducted in inner city areas have found heavy drinkers to be more materially disadvantaged (Weiner *et al.*, 1983).

Diet. Like drinking, diet is not yet well understood. Famine is known to produce babies of low birthweight, of course, with correspondingly high rates of perinatal mortality, but pre-term babies born to obese mothers are also likely to be of low birthweight and to die in infancy (for example, Lucas *et al.*, 1988). Precisely which parts of the mother's diet are the most important is not yet clear (Stein *et al.*, 1975; Schofield, Wheeler and Stewart, 1987). Evidence from intervention studies, for example, suggests that preventing low birthweight by supplementing the mother's diet may not always lead to a reduction in perinatal morbidity and mortality, and methodological problems mean that the effects of diet itself have not always been disentangled from the effects of being given advice and simply receiving attention (Rush, 1982; Bakketeig *et al.*, 1984). It is also important to note that diet interacts with both smoking and drinking in that mothers who smoke or drink may eat different things and different amounts from those who do not, and smoking and drinking may reduce the nutritional benefits for both mother and fetus.

Work. Government statistics show that 70 per cent of married women go out to work (around half of them full-time and half of them part-time) (OPCS, 1991b). Almost 50 per cent of *pregnant* women work and, of those, three-quarters continue even after 30 weeks (Chamberlain, 1984). Considerable interest has been shown in the possible consequences for the baby – less so for the mother and the rest of the family – and reviews of the literature are to be found in papers by Chamberlain and Garcia (1983), Chamberlain (1984), Saurel-Cubizolles *et al.* (1985), and Stein, Susser and Hatch (1986).

Three studies deserve special attention because of their scope and statistical sophistication. The first is by Peters *et al.* (1984), and was based on the 1958 British Perinatal Mortality Survey. All stillbirths and neonatal deaths for March, April and May 1958 were compared with a 'control population' of all live births and stillbirths in the first week of March that year, a total of almost

17,000. Forty per cent of the women worked – most for more than 30 hours a week, 15 per cent for 45 hours or more – and half of them continued for six months or more into the pregnancy. Between mothers who worked and those who did not there was no difference in toxaemia, pre-term delivery or low birthweight. There was, however, a raised incidence of perinatal death among the children of working mothers, and it was found in every social class. The difference was greatest for Classes I and II (31 per 1,000 for working mothers against 25 per 1,000 for non-working mothers), and it was smallest for Classes IV and V (42 per 1,000 against 40 per 1,000), though it is unclear from the report whether the differences reached statistical significance. Developmental measures at the age of seven showed that, for height, head circumference and attainments in arithmetic and reading, the children of mothers whose work had been manual fared less well than those whose mothers had worked in non-manual jobs. The effects remained even when social class, defined by father's occupation, was controlled.

The second study, by Murphy *et al.* (1984), was based on the Cardiff Births Survey. All singleton births to married first-time mothers from Classes I to V were analyzed, a total of over 20,000. Over 75 per cent of the mothers worked, though whether full-time or part-time was not reported, but almost 90 per cent of them had stopped by 29 weeks – a very different pattern from the 1958 data of Peters *et al.* (1984). Those who did not work were more likely to have a history of medical problems, miscarriage and abortion, and were more likely to be married to unemployed men (in all social groupings) but less likely to attend antenatal classes. Two measures showed a significant difference between the working and non-working groups, even after previous adverse medical history was controlled: a raised incidence of pre-term deliveries in the non-working group; and a raised perinatal mortality rate among the non-working mothers of Classes I and II, almost twice that of the working group. The authors concluded that healthy women who were likely to have healthy outcomes to their pregnancies were those who chose or were chosen to work, and the effects of employment were then generally positive in that work leads to social contact, shared information and perhaps more resources. Murphy, however, like Peters, was careful to acknowledge that what is cause and what is effect remains uncertain. Why the woman works, for example, and the consequences for her, may be especially important mediators (Oakley, 1984), but they have received little attention.

The third study of note was carried out in France (INSERM, 1980). Characteristics of employment that were associated with poor perinatal outcome were identified, and they were found to include a long working week, standing rather than sitting during working hours, having few breaks, having a lengthy journey and performing physically exhausting work. Overall, the study again suggested a more favourable outcome for economically active women.

As a final point, it should be noted that the literature has generally failed to take account of the unpaid work that women carry out in the home. Studies of housework (Oakley, 1974) have found that women at home without paid employment do the equivalent of at least a 40-hour week. In the case of women with paid employment, housework is additional. In neither group have the physical effects upon pregnancy outcome been properly considered.

A model of pregnancy outcome

At the start of the chapter, we examined the epidemiology of poor pregnancy outcome, and we found that one particular social input, class, had marked effects. As Illsley and Mitchell (1984) pointed out in their review of research on low birthweight, social class is

> an intellectual and social construct; it has no material form and cannot directly affect the development of the foetus in its uterine environment or cause its premature expulsion, yet its relationship with so many aspects of child and adult illness and death . . . shows that it nevertheless has biological significance. (p. 9)

How that biological significance is turned into observable outcomes has been at the heart of our review. We have examined the essential statistics together with the findings for a range of psychological mediators. Now we present a model to try to piece together some of the relationships (Figure 2.8). It was this particular model – on class and pregnancy outcome – that formed

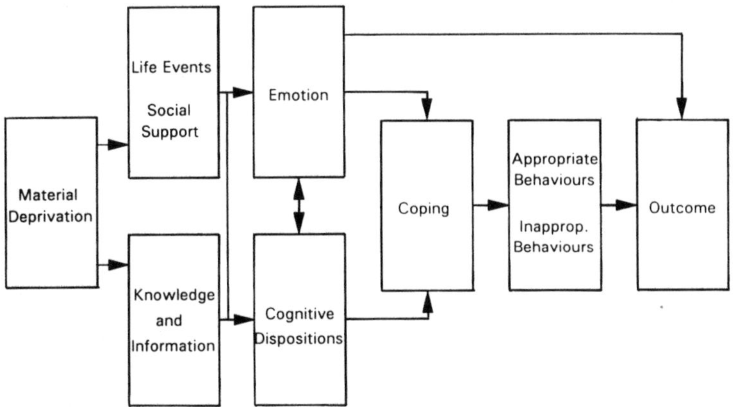

Figure 2.8 A model of psychosocial mediators in pregnancy outcome

the basis of what was to become our general model of health presented in Chapter 1.

The most important aspect of lower social class is probably impoverished material and social conditions and resources, which lead, we suggest, to two principal effects, one an increase in negative life-events and chronic long-term difficulties, often with an absence of social support, the other a reduction in the level of access to information, in part through lack of education. Life-events and lack of support lead in turn to emotional problems, including lowered self-esteem, stress, anxiety, and depression while poor education and lack of access to information produce a corresponding range of cognitive problems, including a lack of knowledge and a set of beliefs and attitudes that lead the woman to see herself as vulnerable to illness and complications but helpless to prevent them. As Bakketeig *et al.* argue: 'the class structure impinges on the distribution of life stresses in two ways: (1) The incidence of potentially negative life-events is greater with descending social class; but (2) resources and skills relevant to coping with such stress are also unevenly distributed, with lower class individuals possessing fewer . . .' (Bakketeig *et al.*, 1984, p. 124). The emotional and cognitive effects combine, we suggest, to produce a set of coping styles and strategies that are characterized by hopelessness and a willingness to take potentially serious risks. From there, it is a short step to inappropriate behaviours and thence to negative outcomes.

As we have noted in Chapter 1, the model is, at present, essentially a framework for integrating past findings and guiding future research. There are many gaps to be filled in the existing body of knowledge and much to be done to establish the strengths and weights of the proposed links and causal pathways. There are three points to note. First, we do not argue that all links between impoverished material and social circumstances are mediated in the ways our model emphasizes. In our discussion of the Black Report in Chapter 1 we distinguished three versions of the material deprivation/culture/behaviour interpretation of social inequalities. The first says that material deprivation causes poor outcomes *directly* (for example, damp housing makes the infant ill). The second says that the link is *indirect* through behaviour (for example, lack of money makes it difficult to pay for travel to antenatal care or for babysitting during clinic visits, and so visits are not made). The third says that material deprivation *produces* the stressful life-events, combined with poor social support and lack of education and knowledge, which lead through behaviours to negative outcomes. All three links are possible.

Our second point concerns the state of the evidence about psychosocial mediators. As we have noted, there are methodological weaknesses in some of the research, and we have tried to weight our discussion accordingly. But sometimes there are straightforward gaps in what is known about the way in which some of the variables we have described are distributed by social class. There is an obvious danger that we may appear to imply that working class is 'bad' and middle class is 'good', but that is not our intention. We may also appear to emphasize cognition unduly, given the present state of the evidence, perhaps at the expense of cultural explanations particularly. In the case of smoking, for example, women may smoke because they do not appreciate the risks (as we suggest), or because smoking buffers their stress (again, as we suggest), or because their culture approves and even encourages the behaviour, although the women know the dangers perfectly well. All three explanations are possible, but the evidence simply does not allow one to weight them at present. Finally, we are aware that our model is oversimplified. The causal pathways are all seen as left-to-right with no allowance for feedback. This is because our main concern has been to draw attention to the mechanisms by which deprivation produces its outcomes.

A programme of research

We come now to our own research on pregnancy outcome. In Chapter 1 we suggested that there are two types of outcome: 'hard' outcomes such as mortality indices, and 'soft' outcomes such as satisfaction with services. The focus of the programme of research we shall report is on one of the 'soft' outcomes, namely satisfaction – with maternity care, with the quality of the birth experience, and with medical communications at the time of the birth. We report three studies. The first is a study of the role of cognitive factors: the importance of the pre-existing knowledge and attitudes of pregnant women as predictors of their satisfaction with maternity care. The second study examines factors associated with women's satisfaction with the birth experience. The third study examines the relative contributions of cognitive and affective variables to satisfaction with medical communications when a child's mental or physical impairment is first diagnosed.

Study I Parents' satisfaction with maternity care: The importance of pre-existing attitudes and knowledge

Research into communications in medicine has produced two recurrent findings: many patients report dissatisfaction with the way their doctors communicate with them; and many doctors complain that their patients fail to comply with their advice and treatment (Fletcher, 1973; Bennett, 1976; Ley, 1988). A number of attempts have been made to account for the findings theoretically, and among the most influential has been the cognitive model of Ley and his colleagues (Ley and Spelman,

1967; Ley, 1982). Satisfaction and compliance, Ley argues, are both dependent upon understanding and memory: if patients understand and remember what they are told, they are more likely to be satisfied with the encounter and in turn to comply with what their doctor suggests (Figure 1.3).

Ley's model has been tested many times, in both correlational and intervention designs, and it has received good support (Ley, 1977, 1982, 1988). There is, however, one important weakness, namely that the model says nothing about what the patient and doctor *bring to* the encounter – the history of their relationship and previous encounters, their expectations about each other, and so on. Of particular importance, it might be thought, are the patient's knowledge and attitudes, for they are likely to have a substantial influence on satisfaction and compliance, both directly in their own right and indirectly through the mediation of comprehension and memory (Figure 2.9).

Knowledge and attitudes provide the focus for our study. What was needed, we believed, was a *prospective* design, in which knowledge and attitudes would be measured at the outset and would be used to predict later satisfaction. The subjects were parents-to-be, and they were examined on three occasions: at the start of a course of antenatal classes towards the end of the pregnancy; at the end of the classes six weeks later; and finally, where possible, shortly after the birth. Knowledge (about medical and hospital services, the later stages of pregnancy, the birth and basic parentcraft) and attitudes (towards medicine and hospital care, the classes, and the birth itself) were measured at

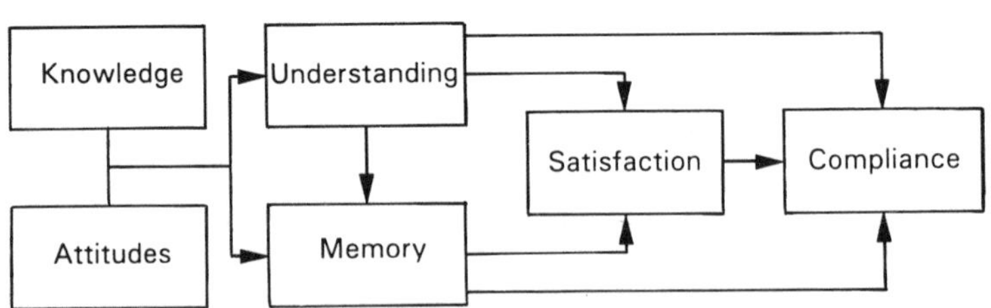

Figure 2.9 Study I: an expanded model of doctor–patient communication

Time 1 and Time 2, and satisfaction with outcome was measured at Time 3. The greater the knowledge and the more positive the attitudes, we predicted, the greater the satisfaction.

Design and procedure

The study was conducted in Canterbury, at the antenatal classes on parentcraft run by the Kent and Canterbury Hospital, which is the district general hospital serving Canterbury and its surroundings. All mothers who register with the hospital for maternity care are invited to a six-week course of classes, and they are encouraged to bring their partner – or their mother or a friend, if they prefer. The classes are held one evening a week, for an hour and a half, and they are organized by the hospital and community midwives. They are designed to provide basic information about the later stages of pregnancy, labour and delivery, hospital services, and infant care and feeding, and also to teach relaxation and breathing.

Two series of classes were included in the study, and all first-time parents-to-be who attended were approached at the first meeting. All 73 who were present agreed to take part, and there were 41 mothers, of whom 32 were accompanied, in each case by the father. Each subject was given a questionnaire to complete during the meeting, and was then followed up with the same questionnaire six weeks later at the final class. Shortly after the birth, a third questionnaire was sent, this time by post. Of the 73 subjects, 48 (66 per cent) were contacted successfully at Time 2 and 29 (60 per cent of the 48) at Time 3. Many of those we failed to see at Time 2 were lost because the classes were so near the end of the pregnancy that the babies had already been delivered.

As part of the first questionnaire, items were included about occupation, so that social class could be determined. Using the father's occupation – or the mother's where the father was not a member of the household – each respondent was classified according to the Standard Occupational Classification (OPCS, 1990), and the six categories were then divided at III non-manual/III manual to give two bands, 'middle-class' and 'working-class'. There were 46 middle-class subjects and 27 working-class subjects. The majority of the middle-class group (32/46) had received a higher education, while the majority of the working-class group (17/27) had not ($chi^2 = 6.1$; df 1; $p < 0.05$).

The questionnaires were designed by ourselves especially for the study. The attitude questionnaire consisted of twenty items, each with a five-point scale from 'Agree' to 'Disagree', scoring from 1 for a negative attitude to 5 for a positive attitude. The items were chosen to tap the areas outlined earlier, and were based in part on the work of Oakley (1977, 1980). The knowledge questionnaire consisted of twenty-five items, to which the respondent answered 'Yes', 'No', or 'Don't know', and scored 0 for an incorrect answer or 'Don't know' and 1 for a correct answer. The items were all concerned with topics that were covered routinely in the classes, and were based on standard texts in midwifery. The satisfaction questionnaire consisted of fifteen questions, each with a five-point scale from 'Dissatisfied' (1) to 'Satisfied' (5).

To simplify our analyses, we first factor analyzed the Time 1 attitude questionnaire, using maximum likelihood factor analysis with Varimax rotation, and three interpretable factors were revealed: 'medicine and hospital care', 'parentcraft classes' and 'childbirth'. Subsequent analyses made use of the factor scores. For knowledge and satisfaction, items were summed to form scales. Cronbach's alpha reliability coefficients were 0.81 for knowledge and 0.69 for satisfaction.

Results

The main purpose of the study was to explore the possible significance of attitudes and knowledge for later satisfaction with outcome, and the data were analyzed by multiple regression. Two analyses were conducted on all respondents combined. The first used knowledge and attitudes at Time 1 as predictors of satisfaction at Time 3, and the second used the corresponding measures at Time 2 as predictors. Both analyses produced significant effects (Table 2.1). At Time 1, 53 per cent of the variance was explained, and there were two significant predictors of satisfaction: attitude to medicine and hospital care, and attitude to childbirth. At Time 2, 31 per cent of the variance was explained, and there was now just one significant predictor: attitude to medicine and hospital care. Knowledge played no part in either of the equations: the one reliable predictor of outcome was attitude to medicine and hospital care.

Table 2.1 Study I: Attitudes and knowledge as predictors of satisfaction: multiple regression analysis

	Beta	R^2
Satisfaction: Time 1 predictors		
Attitude A: Medicine and hospital care	0.57***	
Attitude B: Parentcraft classes	−0.17	
Attitude C: Childbirth	0.41**	
Knowledge	0.09	0.53**
Satisfaction: Time 2 predictors		
Attitude A: Medicine and hospital care	0.42*	
Attitude B: Parentcraft classes	−0.07	
Attitude C: Childbirth	0.27	
Knowledge	0.05	0.31

* $p < 0.05$
** $p < 0.01$
*** $p < 0.001$

Discussion

The immediate implication of our findings, we believe, is that Ley's model should be extended to allow the *mechanisms* by which attitudes influence satisfaction to be explored in detail. There are also two other issues to address, however, and the first concerns the effects of the antenatal classes. Although the classes were associated with a significant increase in knowledge – sometimes from a very low level indeed – there was little effect on attitudes, which might at first seem disappointing. In fact, however, it is not, for an essential way in which people prepare themselves emotionally and intellectually for crises, and develop an internal locus of control for dealing with them, is what has been called 'the work of worrying' (Janis, 1958; Janis and Leventhal, 1965; Doering *et al.*, 1980). The consequences for childbirth are especially important, since 'the work of worrying' helps the woman to gain 'active control', which leads her to a more positive experience of the birth itself, in part because she is more likely to remain conscious and aware (Doering *et al.*, 1980). Static attitudes, or even increased scepticism, may thus be a positive sign.

The second issue concerns the links between inputs and outcomes – the processes that mediate between what the subject brings and the eventual outcome, whether psychological (including satisfaction) or physical (including the health of the mother and baby). The social input we are stressing in this chapter is social class, and the present study revealed important effects: while middle-class parents were more knowledgeable than working-class parents, they had a less positive attitude to medicine and hospital care (Table 2.2). Some of the strongest evidence for class effects in health comes from the statistics on pregnancy, birth, and infancy – yet research on the processes that link class to outcomes has scarcely begun. To draw out those links, we believe, and to integrate them into a theoretical model, continues to be among the most important tasks the literature faces.

Study II Women's satisfaction with the quality of the birth experience

The quality of a woman's childbirth experience is vital both to her well-being and to her future relationship with her partner and child (Doering, Entwisle and Quinlan, 1980). Childbirth has been viewed theoretically as a 'crisis' (especially for first-time mothers) or at least a stressful life-event (Chertok, 1969). Social and psychological resources are thought to mediate the effects of stressful events on well-being. For example, Henneborn and Cogan (1975) and Norr *et al.* (1977) have reported that both preparation for the birth and partner participation have a positive effect upon the quality of childbirth, although the mechanisms that mediate between preparation and quality of childbirth remain an area of inquiry. Similarly, it has been argued that the effect of stressful life-events can be buffered by social support, either by reducing the stress itself or by increasing an individual's coping strategies (Nuckolls, Cassel and Kaplar, 1972; Dimsdale *et al.*, 1979). Other demographic and psychosocial variables the literature suggests may affect the quality of the woman's birth experience include age (Norr *et al.*, 1977; O'Brien and Smith, 1981), social class (Nelson, 1983; McIntosh, 1989), expectations and experience of pain (Norr *et al.*, 1977; Doering, Entwisle and

Table 2.2 Study I: Means for social class

	Middle-class		Working-class			
	Mean	SD	Mean	SD	df	t
Time 1						
Attitude A: Medicine and hospital care	22.6	4.0	26.6	3.4	71	4.4***
Attitude B: Parentcraft classes	13.5	2.3	14.3	1.4	71	1.6
Attitude C: Childbirth	21.1	3.1	21.6	2.7	71	0.7
Knowledge	14.9	4.0	10.7	4.5	71	4.1***
Time 2						
Attitude A: Medicine and hospital care	21.7	4.1	25.8	3.0	46	3.2**
Attitude B: Parentcraft classes	14.0	1.7	14.4	1.2	46	0.7
Attitude C: Childbirth	20.6	2.4	19.7	3.5	46	1.0
Knowledge	18.7	2.2	16.3	3.0	46	3.0**

* $p < 0.05$
** $p < 0.01$
*** $p < 0.001$

Quinlan, 1980), and personal control (Green, Coupland and Kitzinger, 1990), but as yet there has been little attempt to integrate the variables theoretically.

The objective of our second study was to make use of our own model to try to draw together a number of the variables (Quine, Rutter and Gowen, 1993). The study explored the significance of social inputs and social psychological mediators for women's satisfaction with the quality of their birth experience. The social inputs the study highlights are social class and age, and the mediators are social support, preparation, information about childbirth, locus of control, and expectations and experience of pain.

Design and procedure

The study was prospective in design and was again conducted at the Kent and Canterbury Hospital. First-time mothers-to-be were approached at maternity classes at the hospital towards the end of their pregnancies, and all 60 women who were present agreed to take part. Each subject completed a questionnaire during the class and gave permission for the researcher to interview her once the baby had arrived. After the birth the mothers were contacted by telephone and visited in their own homes, where they completed a second questionnaire. Of the 60 subjects only one was not contacted successfully at Time 2. The subjects' ages ranged from 16 to 38.

In the first questionnaire we included items about occupation so that social class could be determined. Using the father's occupation, or the mother's where the father was not a member of the household, each respondent was assigned to one of the usual six categories, which were then divided at III non-manual/ III manual to give two bands, 'middle class' and 'working class'. There were 28 middle-class subjects and 31 working-class subjects.

The questionnaires were designed especially for the study. The preparation questionnaire consisted of four items concerning the woman's preparation for childbirth, each with a five-point scale from 'Strongly disagree' to 'Strongly agree'. At Time 2 the questions were concerned with her views about how prepared she felt she had been. The information questionnaire consisted of four items concerning whether the subject felt she had understood the information given about childbirth, had been given enough information or had thought the information was too technical or too difficult to remember. The pain questionnaire consisted of three items at Time 1 and five at Time 2: at Time 1 we asked whether the subject expected childbirth to be painful and whether she believed that medical staff and breathing exercises would help her to control the pain; and at Time 2 we asked whether childbirth had been more painful than expected and whether the birth had gone as the subject had expected, together with the same items as before about pain control. The support questionnaire consisted of five items which tapped the subject's perceptions of her support from husband, family, friends, neighbours and professional services. Locus of control was measured by the Multidimensional Health Locus of Control Scale (MHLC) (Wallston and Wallston, 1978b), which taps whether the woman believes her health is under the control of herself, powerful others or chance. The outcome measure, satisfaction with the quality of the birth experience, was measured at Time 2. Mothers were asked to rate their satisfaction on a five-point scale from 'Very satisfied' to 'Very dissatisfied'. Two additional outcome measures were also used: a set of nine bipolar items measured on five-point scales which enquired about symptoms of stress (Martin and Roberts, 1984); and a set of items describing the babies' behaviour (feeding, sleeping, crying, etc.), designed by ourselves. The reliabilities of each of the scales (Cronbach's alpha) were computed and ranged from 0.59 to 0.90.

Results

Social class and age. First, we performed a series of univariate analyses to investigate differences in attitudes between the social classes. At Time 1 working-class women felt slightly more prepared for the birth than did middle-class women, though the difference did not reach statistical significance. However, after the birth at Time 2, middle-class women were now significantly more likely to feel that they *had* been prepared. Working-class women were significantly less satisfied with the information given: they were less likely to feel that they had been given enough information, less likely to feel that they had understood what information *had* been given and more likely than middle-class women to describe it as 'too technical'. Middle-class women felt significantly better supported by their partners, family, friends and neighbours than did working-class women. There were also differences in locus of control, in that working-class women were significantly more likely to attribute both health and illness to chance than were middle-class women. Working-class women were on average less satisfied with their birth experience, with a mean figure only just above the mid-point of the scale. There were no effects for expected or reported pain.

Second, we investigated whether there were differences in attitudes between older and younger women. We split the sample into two equal groups: women aged between 16 and 25 and women aged between 26 and 38. There were no differences between the two groups for preparation at Time 1 or Time 2, or for expected or reported pain, or support at Time 1. However, older women felt better informed at Time 1 and better supported at Time 2 than the younger women. Younger women were more likely to attribute their health to chance than were older women.

Predicting quality of the birth experience. The first stage of this part of our analysis was to use hierarchical regression, in which the variables were entered in blocks that represent their assumed causal pathways. The final variance explained was 56 per cent (Figure 2.10). Each block added significantly to the variance accumulated by the preceding blocks, and the greatest increment was for the Time 2 block, which added 38 per cent. In order to provide greater information on the structure of the interrelationships between individual variables and the quality of the women's birth experience, we used path analysis, in which the hierarchical blocks were 'unpacked', and the pathways linking demographic inputs to outcome were traced by means of repeated multiple regression analyses. All the factors from the hierarchical analysis were included, but only those with statistically reliable paths appear in the figure (Figure 2.11). The force of the diagram is the clarity with which the paths are revealed, and there are several points to note. The total variance explained was 53 per cent. Social class affected both social support and information at Time 1: working-class women felt less supported than middle-class women by their partner, family, friends and neighbours, and they felt less informed than middle-class women, were more likely to consider that they had not received sufficient information and

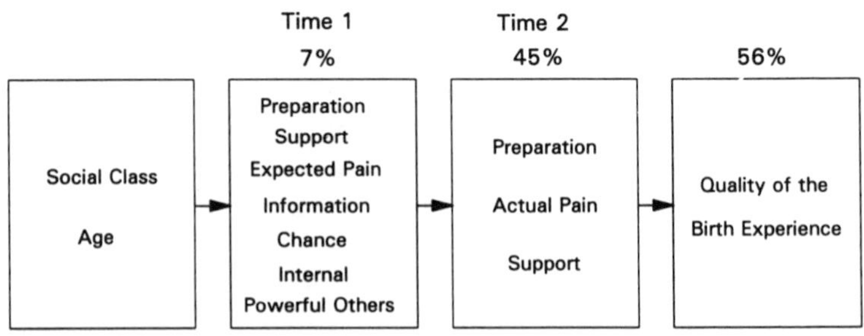

Figure 2.10 Study II: hierarchical analysis for quality of the birth experience

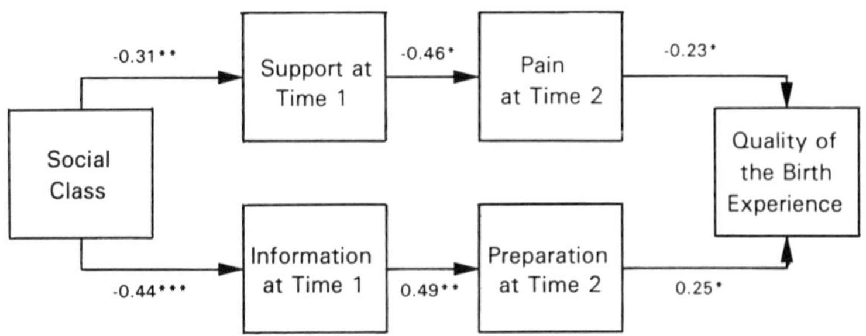

Figure 2.11 Study II: path analysis for quality of the birth experience. Variance explained: 53%. (* $p < 0.05$ ** $p < 0.01$ *** $p < 0.001$)

that the information offered was in any case too technical and too difficult to understand. Women who felt supported at Time 1 reported less pain during the birth than those women who felt that they were not receiving adequate support, and women who felt less pain in turn reported greater satisfaction with the birth experience. Women who felt informed felt more prepared for the birth, and preparation also led to greater satisfaction with the birth experience. Age played no part in the analysis, probably because working-class women tend to have their babies younger. The effects of age are therefore absorbed by social class.

Quality of the birth experience and outcome for mother and baby. Our final analyses concerned the *consequences* of a good or poor birth experience. In order to present as clear a picture as possible, we collapsed the five-point satisfaction scale so that it became a dichotomous variable. The values 'Very satisfied' and 'Satisfied' were combined and the values 'Dissatisfied' and 'Very dissatisfied' were combined, and the middle value was omitted. A series of t-tests were conducted to investigate the relationship between women's satisfaction with the quality of their birth experience and a number of other variables that might be thought to be consequences: each of the stress items from the Martin and Roberts stress scale, and each item from the scale we had used to measure the women's reports of their babies' behaviour.

The results for the stress analysis are shown in Table 2.3. Of the nine items in the scale, six produced statistically significant differences between women who were satisfied and those who were dissatisfied with their birth experience. Women who were satisfied were more even tempered, more self-confident, less depressed, more able to cope with life, more calm and unworried and more healthy than were women who were dissatisfied with the birth experience. The results for the babies' reported behaviour are shown in Table 2.4. Women who were satisfied with the quality of their birth experience were more likely to report that their child was easy to settle to sleep, slept well, was feeding well, did not cry much and was not irritable. Together, the findings thus confirm that the quality of a woman's birth experience may influence her own symptoms of stress and her later perceptions of the baby, but they must be treated with caution: measures of quality of birth experience and mother and baby outcomes were all taken at a single point in time, and the direction of causality cannot be determined.

Table 2.3 Study II: Quality of the birth experience and stress: t-tests

	Satisfied with birth experience		Dissatisfied with birth experience		
Item	Mean	SD	Mean	SD	t
Full of energy	3.0	1.0	2.3	1.1	1.8 N/S
No worries about the future	3.4	1.1	2.9	1.0	1.4 N/S
Even-tempered	3.9	0.9	2.8	1.0	3.5 **
Lots of self-confidence	3.9	0.9	2.8	1.0	3.6 **
Never depressed	4.0	0.9	3.0	1.0	2.8 **
Not losing weight	2.4	1.1	2.9	0.7	1.8 N/S
Able to cope with life	4.1	0.9	2.4	1.1	4.7 ***
Calm and unworried	3.9	1.0	2.6	0.5	5.7 ***
Usually in good health	4.5	0.8	2.8	0.9	5.2 ***
Overall score	33.0	5.0	24.0	5.1	4.9 ***

** $p < 0.01$
*** $p < 0.001$

Table 2.4 Study II: Quality of the birth experience and the child's behaviour: t-tests

	Satisfied with birth experience		Dissatisfied with birth experience		
Item	Mean	SD	Mean	SD	t
Easy to settle to sleep	3.9	1.1	2.6	1.4	2.9 **
Sleeps well	4.4	0.8	2.8	1.4	3.8 **
Feeds well	4.3	1.1	2.8	1.2	3.8 ***
Cries little	4.1	1.0	2.9	1.2	3.0 **
Not irritable	4.1	0.9	2.8	0.8	4.4 ***
Overall score	20.7	3.5	13.8	4.6	4.7 ***

** $p < 0.01$
*** $p < 0.001$

Discussion

The results of this second study demonstrate the importance of both social support and adequate information as *mediators* between social class and the experience of childbirth. Working-class women appear to be disadvantaged in both respects: they are less supported than middle-class women, and they lack adequate information. They are consequently less likely to find childbirth a rewarding experience. Intervention studies in which women have been offered social support during pregnancy and labour typically find that it has positive effects (Sosa *et al.*, 1980; Oakley, 1985; Oakley and Rajan, 1991) – fewer admissions to hospital during pregnancy, shorter labours, greater awareness during delivery, less use of neonatal intensive care by babies, greater health service use by mothers and babies after the birth, greater satisfaction with care and improved psychological well-being, especially reduced anxiety. Oakley and Rajan (1991) observe that the conventional picture of close-knit supportive social networks based on kin and neighbourhood among working-class women reported in studies in the 1950s is not borne out by more recent studies which find that working-class women often lack social support. Women who feel they have adequate information, too, are more likely to feel prepared for the birth and so are more satisfied with the experience. Social class does not have a *direct* effect on outcome; instead it has its effects through social support on the one hand and information on the other.

Study III Breaking the news of severe mental impairment: A study of doctor–parent communication

Our third study concerns parents' satisfaction with medical communications at the time of the birth. The birth of a baby is usually awaited with joyous anticipation, and during the pregnancy the parents develop an idealized picture of their 'perfect' baby (Solnit and Stark, 1961). Most of the 700,000 babies born in England and Wales each year are healthy, and it was with them that our previous two studies were concerned. Three or four per cent, however, have impairments which are present at birth or arise during delivery or immediately afterwards. About four in every thousand babies are born with severe mental impairment. For their parents, dreams of the perfect baby are shattered when they are informed about the baby's condition. How the information is given is the subject of this third study.

There is an extensive literature on the way parents are first informed of a child's diagnosis of severe mental or physical impairment. Several studies have viewed the process as a crisis producing grief, followed by stages of shock and disbelief, denial, anger, adaptation and adjustment, similar to the phases identified in the bereavement literature (Kennedy, 1970; Drotar *et al.*, 1975; Emde and Brown, 1978; Cunningham, 1979). Reference is also made to 'chronic sorrow' (Olshansky, 1962). A number of studies report on the identification of Down's syndrome (Drillien and Wilkinson, 1964; Berg, Gilderdale and Way, 1969; Carr, 1970; Pueschel and Murphy, 1976; Cunningham and Sloper, 1977; Lucas and Lucas, 1980), while others are concerned with congenital malformation such as spina bifida (Hare *et al.*, 1966; D'Arcy, 1968; Fost, 1981) or severe learning difficulties (Hewett, 1972; Smith and Phillips, 1978; Quine and Pahl, 1986, 1987). Evidence suggests that the way parents are told affects both the way in which they adjust to the situation and their early treatment of the child (Brinkworth, 1975; Pugh and Russell, 1977; Svarstad and Lipton, 1977; Springer and Steele, 1980). Most studies document high levels of dissatisfaction among parents with the way they were first informed of the child's handicapping condition – over 70 per cent dissatisfied in some instances – and they describe the parents' reaction to the news. However, there has been little attempt to account for the findings theoretically.

Why are some parents so dissatisfied with the way they were told about their child's impairment, while others speak appreciatively of the understanding way in which the news was broken? Are there common patterns that characterize encounters that parents found satisfactory rather than unsatisfactory? What is good practice in this field, and what can be done do improve communications between parents and professionals when mental and physical impairment are diagnosed? This study considers some of the factors associated with satisfaction with medical communications at the time of diagnosis, and tests two competing social psychological models which have been used in other studies to account for parental/patient satisfaction. We shall be concerned with only the parents' point of view, which means that we shall be investigating not what 'really' happened, but what the parents considered to have happened. The discussion draws its evidence from a study of 178 families caring for children with severe learning disabilities.

Models of doctor–patient communication

Ley's cognitive model. Among the most influential models of doctor–patient communication has been the cognitive model of Ley and his colleagues (Ley and Spelman, 1967; Ley, 1977, 1988), as we saw in Chapter 1 and also earlier in this present chapter. Ley argues that, for communication to be effective, the message it contains must be understood and remembered. Patients' failures to understand stem from three interrelated problems: the material presented to them is often too difficult to understand; patients often lack elementary technical medical knowledge; and they often have active misconceptions which militate against proper understanding. Failure to understand and remember leads to dissatisfaction and failure to comply with advice and instructions. In a series of intervention studies Ley and his colleagues were able to increase patient satisfaction with communication by increasing understanding and memory (Ley *et al.*, 1976a; Ley *et al.*, 1976b; Ley, 1977), suggesting that the model is valuable both for theory and for practice.

Korsch's affective model. A second important model comes from Korsch, Gozzi and Francis (1968). In a major study of 800 consultations at a paediatric clinic at a children's hospital in Los Angeles, Korsch and her colleagues showed that satisfaction with the medical encounter was related to three parental ratings of the doctor's affective behaviour: being friendly rather than business-like; seeming to understand the mother's concern rather than not understanding; and being a good rather than a poor communicator. Korsch believes that if these essential ingredients are missing from doctor–patient/parent interaction, patients/parents will be dissatisfied. While Ley focuses on cognition, therefore, Korsch is concerned with affect and social interaction.

Design and procedure

Our own study investigates families caring for children with severe learning disabilities in two health districts in the South East of England (Quine and Rutter, 1993). The study had two stages. In the first stage 399 children up to 16 years of age who had been or were likely to be assessed as suitable for education in a special school were seen by the research team. The children were assessed using the Disability Assessment Schedule developed by Holmes, Shah and Wing (1982). The DAS collects information from the teacher or care assistant who knows each child best about the child's mobility, confidence, self-help skills, vision, hearing, communication skills, behaviour problems and medical conditions. At the second stage, interviews were carried out with the carers of a stratified random sample of children, using a structured questionnaire. The sample was chosen with proportional allocation for age and sex so that it matched the population from which it was drawn.

The parents were asked a number of questions about the way the news of the child's condition was broken to them: how old the child was when the diagnosis was confirmed; for how long they had been anxious about the child before being given a diagnosis; how satisfied they were with the way the news had been given. They were also asked to rate the doctor's behaviour on five bipolar items, like those of Korsch, measured on five-point scales. These included whether the doctor had a sympathetic manner; whether he understood the mother's concern; and whether he was direct, approachable and a good communicator. Finally, in line with Ley, parents were asked to rate their understanding and memory of the information they received, on a series of five-point scales. These items included ratings of whether they understood the information, remembered it, found it not too technical and felt that they had received sufficient information.

The great majority of the children were living with their natural mother and father and with other children. Single-parent families made up 13 per cent of the total, and most of these were mothers living with their children. In 54 per cent of families the handicapped child was the youngest in the family, while in 35 per cent he or she was the eldest; 18 per cent of the sample were the only child in the family. In 166 cases the chief carer was the child's mother. Twelve children were fostered or in residential care and we excluded them since family data were not available. Our analyses are therefore based on 166 cases.

The diagnoses of the children are shown in Figure 2.12. Thirty

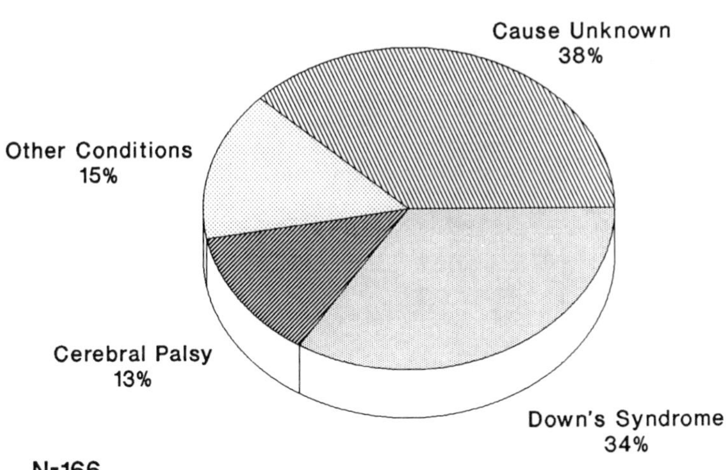

Figure 2.12 Study III: diagnostic category

per cent of the children had Down's syndrome, 13 per cent had cerebral palsy, and 15 per cent had other known conditions such as primary genetic or chromosomal abnormalities, metabolic disorders, developmental defects such as spina bifida, brain damage caused by accident or illness, or fetal rubella syndrome. Thirty-eight per cent had severe learning difficulties of unknown cause. A large proportion of the children were quite severely impaired (Figure 2.13). Almost one third were unable to walk by themselves, over one third were unable to feed themselves, one fifth were blind or partially sighted, one third suffered from epileptic fits, and almost half had one or more serious behaviour problems.

Results

When parents were informed. Parents were asked when they were first informed of the diagnosis of mental impairment. The results showed that the parents of 35 per cent of the children were told at birth, 31 per cent during the first year of the child's life, 15 per cent during the second year and 19 per cent during the child's third year or later. Almost three-quarters of parents were told

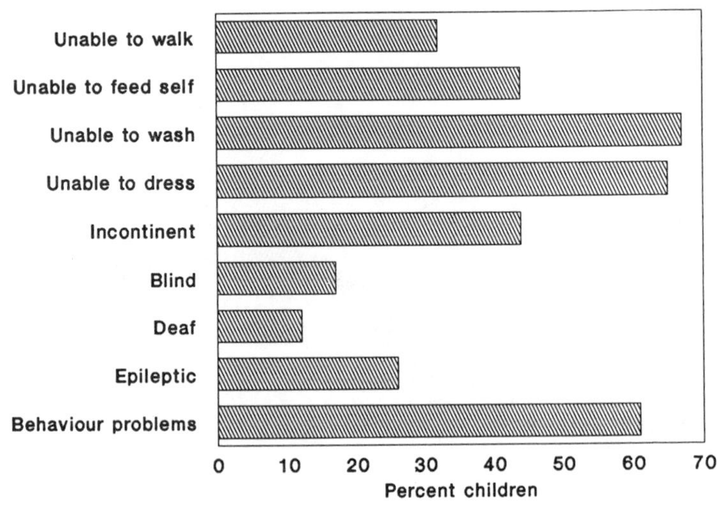

Figure 2.13 Study III: children's impairments

the news by a hospital doctor. In some cases the doctor involved was summoned soon after the birth by the midwifery staff who had delivered the baby. In others it was the paediatrician to whom the child had been referred once developmental delay or other problems had been noted at the clinic. Although some parents were not informed about their child's impairment immediately, some were of course unaware of it or became only slowly aware that something was wrong. Though 35 per cent of parents had known immediately after the birth, almost 30 per cent had been worried about the child for up to one year, 14 per cent had been worried for almost two years, 7 per cent for three years and 7 per cent for nearly four. Four per cent of children had been impaired by accident or illness during childhood, and 3 per cent of parents were unaware of any problems until they were told.

How the news was broken. Parents were asked to recall what they had been told. Sixty-four per cent had been given a (sometimes brief) explanation of the impairment. Twenty-one per cent had been given only a diagnosis. In only 27 per cent of cases had opinions as to future development or advice on how to help and manage the child been given. Many commented on the difficulty of the task for doctors, but many were critical of the blunt way in which the news had been given. One parent, for example, told us: 'I didn't notice anything about her features – she had tremendous feeding problems. Eventually I complained and was immediately transferred to X hospital. Nothing had been said. The houseman asked me, "Do you know why you are here?" I said that the baby had feeding problems. An hour later the paediatrician and his entourage came in. He asked if I'd noticed anything different about her. I said, "No." The houseman then told me that she was a mongol. Later he came in with a book with a picture of a woman with Down's syndrome, which he tossed onto the bed. He said, "That's what she'll look like." It was an old-fashioned picture of an institutionalized person – I was terribly upset.'

Parents were sometimes faced with delay, denial and evasion at the hospital. Sometimes newborn babies were taken away to special care nurseries without explanation. Some mothers did not see their babies again for three or four days. One mother of a child with cerebral palsy told us: 'They wouldn't let me see her until the following day. By that time my fears of what she would be like were far worse than if I'd seen her straight away.' The problem was often compounded by changes in the hospital routine or the reactions of the staff which alerted parents' suspicions: 'I knew immediately that something was wrong, the minute she was born. They all gathered round to look at her. Then they wrapped her up and took her away. I kept asking: "Is she all right?" and they would say: "Yes, she's fine, don't worry." But they must have realized I knew, so why didn't they tell me the truth straight away?'

Parents of children whose impairment was not obvious at birth, or who had emergent handicapping conditions, often had a long period of anxiety and uncertainty before a firm diagnosis was made. Many in this group felt that they had received inadequate and confusing information about the child's condition. Three children had even started at normal school and later been transferred to special schools, though the mothers of two of them had believed that their child was developing perfectly normally. A number of the parents, however, had been the first to recognize that their child was not developing normally. Often they believed that their anxieties about their child's development had been disregarded by professionals. One parent told us: 'The doctor said he just had a feeding problem. We found an article which seemed to describe his condition. We took this to the hospital and insisted on further blood tests. After this a firm diagnosis was made.' The child was found to be suffering from infantile hypercalcaemia.

Reasons for parental dissatisfaction. The timing and nature of the communication we have outlined would lead one to expect high levels of dissatisfaction among parents with the way they were first told about the child's impairment. In fact, 58 per cent reported dissatisfaction, while 33 per cent were satisfied and 9 per cent were unsure. One explanation for parental dissatisfaction frequently cited by medical professionals is that satisfaction is determined by internal factors, by the psychology and personality of the mother, which might lead to a general attitude of dissatisfaction with services. However, there was no correlation in our data between general satisfaction with services and satisfaction with learning about the impairment. Nor was there a significant association between the mother's stress rating on the Malaise Inventory (Rutter, Tizard and Whitmore, 1970) and satisfaction with learning about the impairment. There was, however, a straightforward association between timing and satisfaction (Table 2.5): parents who found out early in the child's life were more satisfied with the way they were told than were those who found out later.

Testing the models of doctor–parent communication. The first stage of our analysis of the two theoretical models was to factor analyze the nine cognition and affect items together, using maximum likelihood factor analysis with Varimax rotation. The result was a two-factor solution which corresponded exactly to the two concepts of affective and cognitive behaviour hypothesized by Korsch and Ley. The affect factor accounted for 46 per cent of the variance, the cognition factor 21 per cent. Each set of items was therefore summed to form a scale, and the reliabilities were computed. Cronbach's alpha was 0.88 for the affect scale and 0.77 for the cognition scale.

The second stage of the analysis was to predict satisfaction by means of stepwise multiple regression. In a first analysis, only the two scales, cognition and affect, were entered in order to

Table 2.5 Study III: Satisfaction with the way the first information was given by age of the children when impairment was diagnosed

	Parents were told		
	At birth (%)	First year (%)	Second year or later (%)
Parents were:			
Satisfied	51	33	27.5
Not satisfied	49	67	72.5
Total	100	100	100
Number	58	52	56

Chi^2 7.6, df 2, $p < 0.05$

examine whether the Korsch model or the Ley model predicted the greater variance. In a second analysis, a number of other variables were added: the age of the child; the age of the child when the parents were first informed of the diagnosis; the diagnosis made; the length of time that parents had worried that the child might have an impairment; and the social class of the family. The results of the first analysis (Table 2.6) showed that the affect scale entered the equation first, explaining 35.7 per cent of the variance. The cognition scale entered second, explaining a further 1.4 per cent of the variance, and confirming that the more important predictor of parental satisfaction was the doctor's affective behaviour. The results of the second analysis (Table 2.7) showed that six variables entered the equation, together explaining 40.1 per cent of the variance. The affect scale again entered first, followed by the cognition scale, age of the child, age of the child when the parents were first informed of the diagnosis, time between first feeling anxious and confirmation of diagnosis, and social class. In both analyses, therefore, Korsch's affect factor was a much stronger predictor of satisfaction than was Ley's cognition factor and the variance added by other predictors was relatively small.

Tracing the paths of mediation. The only social input to play a significant part in the regression analysis was social class, and our final task was to try to trace the paths of mediation from class to satisfaction. The technique we used was path analysis, based on our

Table 2.6 Study III: Satisfaction with the medical encounter by perceptions of cognition and affect: stepwise multiple regression analysis

Step variable entered	% of variance explained	Addition to % variance	Significance of beta in final equation
1. Affect scale	35.7	35.7	***
2. Cognition scale	37.1	1.4	*

F 43.8, df 2, 136, $p < 0.001$
* $p < 0.05$
*** $p < 0.001$

Table 2.7 Study III: Satisfaction with the medical encounter by family and child variables: stepwise multiple regression analysis

Step variable entered	% of variance explained	Addition to % variance	Significance of beta in final equation
1. Affect scale	35.7	35.7	***
2. Cognition scale	37.1	1.4	*
3. Age of child	37.8	0.6	N/S
4. Age of child when parent told of diagnosis	38.3	0.5	*
5. Time between anxiety and confirmation	39.9	1.6	*
6. Social class	40.1	0.2	*

F = 21.2, df 5,160, $p < 0.001$
* $p < 0.05$
*** $p < 0.001$

repeated multiple regression analyses (Figure 2.14). All the variables from the second multiple regression analysis were included, but only those with statistically reliable paths appear in the figure. There are several points to note. The total variance explained was almost 40 per cent. Social class did not have a direct effect on satisfaction, but worked through cognition. Working-class mothers were more likely than middle-class mothers to feel that they had not received sufficient information, that the information they *had* received was too technical, and that it had been too difficult to understand and remember. There was also a *direct* effect of cognition on satisfaction: the more mothers understood and remembered, the more satisfied they were. Much the strongest predictor of satisfaction, however, was affect, as the multiple regression analyses had already indicated: the more positively parents rated the doctor's affective behaviour, the more satisfied they were with the encounter overall. Two other variables to emerge were the age of the child when the parent was informed of the diagnosis and the length of the period of anxiety before it was confirmed: parents who were told earlier in the child's life were more satisfied, as were those who had

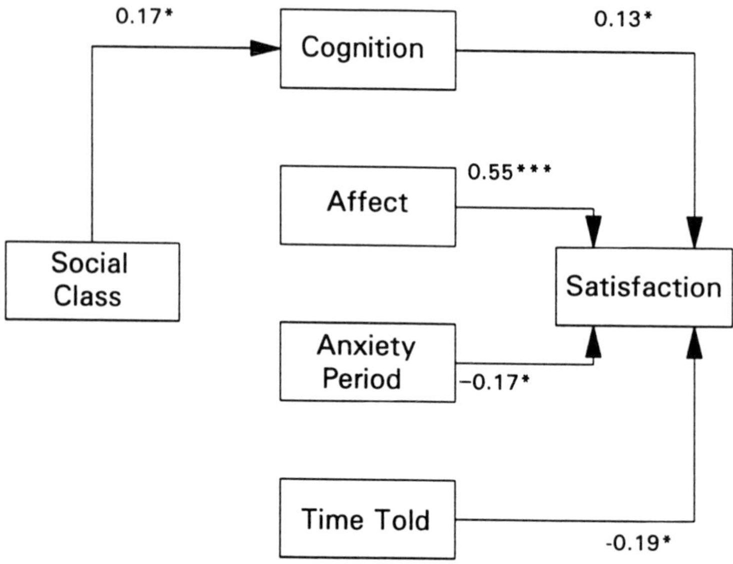

Figure 2.14 Study III: path model of satisfaction with doctor–parent communication. Variance explained: 39.5%. (* $p < 0.05$ *** $p < 0.001$)

worried for a shorter period. Like affect, neither variable was influenced by social class.

Discussion

Our study indicates that there are three main components of satisfaction with the way the news of impairment is given. The first is that parents want to know as soon as possible that something is wrong, even though doctors may be unsure of the exact nature of the impairment. Most studies lead to the conclusion that delay and uncertainty are likely to cause additional distress for the parents and have a lasting effect on their relationship with doctors (Hewett, Newson and Newson, 1970; Gayton and Walker, 1974; Carr, 1975, 1976; Pueschel and Murphy, 1976; Cunningham and Sloper, 1977). Both the National Association for Mental Health (1971) and the Association of Professions for the Mentally Handicapped (APMH)

(1981) have drawn up guidelines for telling parents. APMH recommends that the person to break the news should be the paediatrician, and that the parents should be informed together. In our own study, one parent was often told alone and left to inform the other, and parents found this unsatisfactory. APMH suggests that a written report be given to parents after the initial interview, summarizing what the paediatrician has said and giving details of future sources of help, including the name and telephone number of the parents' key worker.

The second component of satisfaction is a feeling that the person who communicated the information had a sympathetic approach. Korsch, Gozzi and Francis (1968) have reported similar findings, and other studies have confirmed that the doctor's affective behaviour is an important ingredient in medical encounters (Greene, Weinberger and Mamlin, 1980; Ben-Sira, 1984; Stewart, 1984). Our own findings add strong support for Korsch's model.

The third component of satisfaction is information and the part that sharing it can play in reducing anxiety. A large number of parents in our study said that it had been hard to get information about their child's condition, and 74 per cent said they wanted more. Many studies confirm that patients/parents do want information (see the reviews by Cartwright, 1964; Ley and Spelman, 1967; Ley, 1988), even if the illness is cancer, for example, or the patient is dying. Published surveys of satisfaction with hospital and general practice care alike frequently show high levels of dissatisfaction with information, even when patients are satisfied with most other aspects of their care (Ley, 1988). Our own findings confirm the significance of information in this new area, and offer further support to Ley's cognitive model. It is important to remember, however, that the doctor's affective behaviour played a more important role still.

Conclusion: implications for theory, policy and practice

In the final section of the chapter we discuss the implications of our research findings for theory, policy and practice. The implications for theory concern the importance of psychosocial variables in predicting pregnancy outcomes, their role as mediators between socio-demographic factors and outcomes, and the particular importance of social class as an input. The results for policy and practice concern the importance of provision of adequate information about both pregnancy and childhood illness by medical staff, the provision of social support during pregnancy, and the organization of services to advise and support parents who care for children with impairments.

Implications for theory

The first theoretical implication from our programme of research is that social psychological factors have an important role in the prediction of pregnancy outcomes. First, pre-existing attitudes of women towards childbirth, medicine and hospital care are important predictors of satisfaction with maternity care. Second, information and social support, perceptions of preparation, and pain are important predictors of the quality of the birth experience. Women who felt supported experienced less pain, and women who were informed about childbirth felt more prepared for the birth. Third, both cognitive variables concerned with understanding and remembering information about a child's impairment, and measures of the doctor's affective behaviour, are important predictors of satisfaction with the medical encounter at the time when mental or physical impairment is first diagnosed. In all three of our studies, social psychological variables play an important and reliable role in predicting health outcome.

The second implication of our research findings concerns the importance of psychosocial variables as *mediators* between social inputs and outcomes. We have outlined such an approach in Chapter 1. Our three studies suggest that social inputs such as social class, marital status and age achieve their effects on health outcomes partly through social psychological factors such as attitudes, social support and access to information. As Study III has shown, there is no direct link between social class and satisfaction with the medical encounter at the time when a child's mental impairment is diagnosed. Social class in itself does not determine whether the parent will be satisfied with the encounter.

Rather, social class works through cognition: working-class mothers find the information given to them inadequate in a number of ways, and it is this perception of the inadequacy of information that affects satisfaction. Thus, our approach is able to explain *why* social class is a predictor of satisfaction, and this knowledge is useful, of course, both for theory and for policy and practice.

Implications for policy and practice

The first implication for policy and practice concerns the importance of providing adequate, clear information both to women during pregnancy and to parents of children with impairments. Our studies show that it is working-class women in particular who are dissatisfied with the information they receive, and the findings indicate a need to train health professionals to improve their communications. Research in other settings has offered useful explanations of the failure of doctor–patient communication and has indicated how the difficulties can be overcome. Rutter and Maguire (1976) and Rutter (1980), for example, have shown that it is possible to train medical students in communication skills. Ley (1982) has shown that it is possible to improve patients' understanding and recall of information. More radical experiments have involved giving patients open access to their case records (Golodetz, Ruess and Machaus, 1976; Stevens, Staff and MacKay, 1977), providing access to taped information about the illness and its treatment (Midgley and MacRae, 1971), and providing written information in addition to orally presented information (Ellis *et al.*, 1979). A further method of improving communication is patient activation, which covers a number of techniques for encouraging the patient to be more demanding in the doctor–patient interaction (Roter, 1977).

The second implication of our findings concerns the provision of social support during pregnancy. A number of studies have found that intervening to increase support during both pregnancy and labour and delivery has positive effects (Sosa *et al.*, 1980; Oakley *et al.*, 1990). Our own studies suggest that working-class women in particular would benefit.

The final implication of our research for policy and practice concerns the organization of services to advise and support parents who give birth to a child with impairments. We have discussed a number of implications at some length in our earlier work (Quine and Pahl, 1986, 1987), and four in particular stand out: (1) Parents want to be told as early as possible if there is cause for concern about the child, even though doctors may be unsure of the exact nature of the child's impairment. Parents of children with non-specific learning disabilities are particularly vulnerable in this respect. Parents who are told late tend to be dissatisfied. (2) Parents value a sympathetic and caring approach by doctors and other medical staff. (3) Parents want to be given full information about the child's condition. This should not be trusted to memory; parents should be given a written diagnosis and fact sheets about the impairment where possible. (4) Parents are often too distressed at the initial interview to assimilate information. Regular follow-up visits are vitally important. They should be carried out in the parents' home, by a key worker or specialist health visitor who has been appointed to advise the family and help them to negotiate encounters with other professionals.

References

Abel E L (1984), Smoking and pregnancy, *Journal of Psychoactive Drugs*, 16, 327–58.

Alberman E, Benson J and Kani W (1985), Disabilities in survivors of low birthweight, *Archives of Disease in Childhood*, 60, 913–19.

Antonovsky A (1979), *Health, Stress and Coping*, London: Jossey-Bass.

Association of Professions for the Mentally Handicapped (1981), *Team Work in Mental Handicap*, Report of a Conference held on 4th February at Aylesbury.

Bakketeig L S, Hoffman H J and Oakley A R (1984), Perinatal mortality. In M B Bracken (Ed.) *Perinatal Epidemiology*, Oxford: Oxford University Press.

Barnett B and Parker G (1985), Professional and non-professional intervention for highly anxious primiparous mothers, *British Journal of Psychiatry*, 146, 287–93.

Barrison I G, Waterson E J and Murray-Lyon I M (1985), Adverse effects of alcohol in pregnancy, *British Journal of Addiction*, 80, 11–12.

Barrison I G and Wright J T (1984), Moderate drinking during pregnancy and foetal outcome, *Alcohol and Alcoholism*, 19, 167–72.

Beck N C, Siegel L J, Davidson N P, Kormeier S, Breitenstein A and Hall D G (1980), The prediction of pregnancy outcome: maternal preparation, anxiety and attitudinal sets, *Journal of Psychosomatic Research*, 24, 343–51.

Becker M H (1976), Socio-behavioural determinants of compliance. In D L Sackett and R D Haynes (Eds.) *Compliance with Therapeutic Regimens*, Baltimore: Johns Hopkins University Press, 40–50.

Ben-Sira Z (1984), Chronic illness, stress and coping, *Social Science and Medicine*, 18, 725–36.

Bennett A E (1976), *Communication Between Doctors and Patients*, Oxford: Oxford University Press.

Berg J M, Gilderdale S and Way J (1969), On telling the parents of a diagnosis of mongolism, *British Journal of Psychiatry*, 115, 1195–6.

Blau A, Slaff B, Easton K, Welkowitz J, Springarn J and Cohen J (1963), The psychogenic etiology of premature births, *Psychosomatic Medicine*, 25, 201.

Blaxter M (1985), Self-definition of health status and consulting rates in primary care, *Quarterly Journal of Social Affairs*, 1, 131–71.

Blaxter M (1987), Evidence of inequality in health from a national survey, *Lancet*, 4 July, 30–3.

Blaxter M and Paterson E (1982), *Mothers and Daughters: a three-generational study of health attitudes and behaviour*, London: Heinemann.

Blomberg S (1980), Influence of maternal distress during pregnancy on complications in pregnancy and delivery, *Acta Psychiatrica Scandinavica*, 62, 399–404.

Brinkworth R (1975), The unfinished child: early treatment and training for the infant with Down's syndrome, *Journal of the Royal Society of Health*, 2, 73.

Brooke O G, Anderson H R, Bland J M, Peacock J L and Stewart C M (1989), Effects on birthweight of smoking, alcohol, caffeine, socio-economic factors and psychosocial stress, *British Medical Journal*, 298, 795–801.

Brown G W and Harris T (1978), *Social Origins of Depression: A Study of Psychiatric Disorder in Women*, London: Tavistock.

Butler N (1969), *Perinatal Problems*, Second Report, Perinatal Mortality Survey, Edinburgh: Livingstone.

Carr J (1970), Mongolism: telling the parents, *Developmental Medicine and Child Neurology*, 12, 213–21.

Carr J (1975), *Young Children with Down's Syndrome*, London: Butterworth.

Carr J (1976), Effect on the family of a child with Down's syndrome, *Physiotherapy*, 62, 20–4.

Carr-Hill R A (1987), When is a data set complete? A squirrel with a vacuum cleaner, *Social Science and Medicine*, 25, 753–64.

Cartwright A (1964), *Human Relations and Hospital Care*, London: Routledge & Kegan Paul.

Cartwright A (1979), *The Dignity of Labour? A Study of Childbearing and Induction*, London: Tavistock.

Cavenagh A J M, Philips K M, Sheridan B and Williams E M J (1984), Contribution of isolated general practitioner maternity units, *British Medical Journal*, 288, 1438–40.

Chalmers B (1982), Psychological aspects of pregnancy: some thoughts for the eighties, *Social Science and Medicine*, 16, 323–31.

Chalmers B (1983), Psychosocial factors and obstetric complications, *Psychological Medicine*, 13, 333–9.

Chalmers B (1984), Behavioural associations of pregnancy complications, *Journal of Psychosomatic Obstetrics and Gynaecology*, 3, 27–35.

Chalmers I (1984), Innovation in antenatal care – theory and practice, *Journal of the Royal Society of Medicine*, 77, 340–2.

Chamberlain G (1984), *Pregnant Women at Work*, London: Royal Society of Medicine, Macmillan.

Chamberlain G and Garcia J (1983), Pregnant women at work, *Lancet*, January 29, 228–30.

Chertok L (1969), *Motherhood and Personality*, London: Tavistock.

Chertok L (1972), The psychopathology of vomiting of pregnancy. In J Howells (Ed.) *Modern Perspectives in Psycho-obstetrics*, Edinburgh: Oliver and Boyd, 269–82.

Cobb S (1976), Social support as a moderator of life stress, Presidential address to American Psychosomatic Society, 1976, *Psychosomatic Medicine*, 38, 300–14.

Cunningham C (1979), Parent counselling. In M Craft (Ed.) *Tredgold's Mental Retardation, 12th Edition*, London: Baillière Tindall, 313–18.

Cunningham C and Sloper P (1977), Parents of Down's syndrome babies: their early needs, *Child: Care, Health and Development*, 3, 325–48.

D'Arcy F (1968), Congenital defects: mothers' reaction to first information, *British Medical Journal*, 3, 796–8.

Dean A and Lin N (1977), The stress-buffering role of social support: problems and prospects for systematic investigation, *Journal of Nervous and Mental Disease*, 165, 403–17.

Dimsdale J E, Eckenrode J, Haggerty R J, Kaplan B H, Cohen F and Dornbusch S (1979), The role of social support in medical care, *Social Psychiatry*, 14, 175–80.

Doering S G and Entwisle, D R (1975), Preparation during pregnancy and ability to cope with labour and delivery, *American Journal of Orthopsychiatry*, 45, 825–37.

Doering S G, Entwisle D R and Quinlan D (1980), Modeling the quality of women's birth experience, *Journal of Health and Social Behaviour*, 21, 12–21.

Donovan J W (1977), Randomized controlled trial of anti-smoking advice in pregnancy, *British Journal of Preventive and Social Medicine*, 31, 6–12.

Drillien C M and Wilkinson E M (1964), Mongolism: when should parents be told?, *British Medical Journal*, 2, 1306–7.

Drotar D, Baskiewicz A, Irvin N, Kennell J and Klaus M (1975), The adaptation of parents to the birth of an infant with a congenital malformation: a hypothetical model, *Pediatrics*, 56, 710–17.

Elbourne D, Pritchard C and Daurncey M (1986), Perinatal outcomes and related factors: social class differences within and between geographical areas, *Journal of Epidemiology and Community Health*, 40, 301–8.

Ellis D A, Hopkin J, Leitch A G and Crofton J (1979), Doctors' orders: controlled trial of supplementary written information for patients, *British Medical Journal*, 1, 456.

Emde R and Brown C (1978), Adaptation to the birth of a Down's syndrome infant: grieving and maternal attachment, *Journal of the American Academy of Child Psychiatry*, 17, 299–323.

Enkin M (1982), Antenatal classes. In M Enkin and I Chambers (Eds.) *Effectiveness and Satisfaction in Antenatal Care*. London: Spastics International Medical Publications.

Fedrick J and Anderson A (1976), Factors associated with spontaneous preterm birth, *British Journal of Obstetrics and Gynaecology*, 83, 342–50.

Fishbein M and Ajzen I (1975), *Belief, Attitude, Intention and Behaviour*, Reading, Mass: Addison-Wesley.

Fletcher C M (1973), *Communication in Medicine*. London: Nuffield Provincial Hospitals Trust.

Fost N (1981), Counseling families who have a child with a severe congenital anomaly, *Pediatrics*, 67, 321–25.

Fox A J (1988), Social network interaction: new jargon in health inequalities, *British Medical Journal*, 297, 373–4.

Froggatt P (1988), *Fourth Report of the Independent Scientific Committee on Smoking and Health*, DHSS Report, London: HMSO.

Gayton W F and Walker L (1974), Down's syndrome: informing the parents, *American Journal of Diseases of Children*, 127, 510–12.

Godin G and LePage L (1988), Understanding the intentions of pregnant nullipara not to smoke cigarettes after childbirth, *Journal of Drug Education*, 18, 115–24.

Golodetz A, Ruess J and Machaus R L (1976), The right to know: giving the patient his medical record, *Archives of Physical and Medical Rehabilitation*, 57, 78–81.

Graham H (1976), Smoking in pregnancy: the attitudes of expectant mothers, *Social Science and Medicine*, 10, 399–405.

Graham H (1984), *Women, Health and the Family*, Brighton: Wheatsheaf.

Graham H and McKee L (1979), *The First Months of Motherhood:* Vol. 4, *Medical Care. Report on a Health Education Council Project*, University of York.

Green J, Coupland V and Kitzinger J (1990), Expectations, experiences, and psychological outcomes of childbirth: a prospective study of 825 women, *Birth*, 17, 15–24.

Greenberg R S (1983), The impact of prenatal care in different social groups, *American Journal of Obstetrics and Gynecology*, 45, 797–801.

Greene J T, Weinberger M and Mamlin J (1980), Patient attitudes towards health care: expectations of primary care in a clinical setting, *Social Science and Medicine*, 14A, 133–8.

Grimm E R (1967), Psychological and social factors in pregnancy. In S A Richardson and A F Guttmacher (Eds.) *Delivery and Outcome in Childbearing: Its Social and Psychological Aspects*, Baltimore: Williams and Wilkins, 1–52.

Grisso J A, Roman E, Inskip H, Beral V and Donovan J (1984), Alcohol consumption and outcome of pregnancy, *Journal of Epidemiology and Community Health*, 38, 232–5.

Hare E H, Laurence K, Payne H and Rawnsley K (1966), Spina bifida cystica and family stress, *British Medical Journal*, 2, 757–60.

Henderson S, Byrne D G and Duncan-Jones P (1981), *Neurosis and the Social Environment*, Sydney: Academic Press.

Henneborn W J and Cogan R (1975), The effect of husband participation on reported pain and probability of medication during labour and birth, *Journal of Psychosomatic Research*, 19, 215–22.

Hewett S (1972), *The Need for Long Term Care. Institute of Research into Mental Retardation Occasional Papers 2, 3 and 4*, London: Butterworth.

Hewett S, Newson J and Newson E (1970), *The Family and the Handicapped Child*, London: George Allen & Unwin.

Hofmeyer G J, Nikodem V C, Wolman W L, Chalmers B E and Kramer T (1991), Companionship to modify the clinical birth environment: effects on progress and perceptions of labour, and breastfeeding, *British Journal of Obstetrics and Gynaecology*, 98, 756–64.

Holmes N, Shah A and Wing L (1982), The Disability Assessment Schedule: a brief screening device for use with the mentally retarded, *Psychological Medicine*, 12, 879–90.

Howe G, Westhoff C, Vessey M and Yeates D (1985), Effects of age, cigarette smoking and other factors on fertility in a large prospective study, *British Medical Journal*, 290, 1697–700.

Hubert J (1974), Belief and reality: social factors in pregnancy and childbirth. In M P M Richards (Ed.) *The Integration of the Child into a Social World*, Cambridge: Cambridge University Press.

Illsley R and Mitchell R G (Eds.) (1984), *Low Birthweight: A Medical, Psychological and Social Study*, Chichester: Wiley.

INSERM (Institut National de la Santé et de la Recherche Médicale) (1980), Service de presse information. Grossesse et environnement. *Medicine et Hygiène*, 38, 2409–26.

Janis I L (1958), *Psychological Stress*, New York: Wiley.

Janis I L and Leventhal H (1965), Psychological aspects of physical illness and hospital care. In B B Wolman (Ed.) *Handbook of Clinical Psychology*, New York: McGraw-Hill, 1360–77.

Janz N K and Becker M H (1984), The Health Belief Model: A decade later, *Health Education Quarterly*, 11(1), 1–47.

Kapp F T, Horstein S and Graham U (1963), Some psychological factors in prolonged labour due to inefficient uterine action, *Comprehensive Psychiatry*, 4, 9–14.

Kennedy J F (1970), Maternal reactions to the birth of a defective baby, *Social Casework*, 51, 411–16.

Klaus M, Kennell J, Robertson S and Sosa R (1986), Effects of social support during parturition on maternal and infant mortality, *British Medical Journal*, 293, 585–7.

Korsch B, Gozzi E and Francis V (1968), Gaps in doctor–patient communication. I: Doctor–patient interaction and patient satisfaction, *Pediatrics*, 42, 855–71.

Lazarus R S, Averill J R and Opton E M (1974), The psychology of coping: issues of research and assessment. In G V Coehio, D A Hamburg and J E Adams (Eds.), *Coping and Adaptation*, New York: Basic Books.

Lederman R, Lederman E, Work B and McCann D A (1978), The relationship of maternal anxiety, plasma catecholamines and plasma cortisol to progress in labour, *American Journal of Obstetrics and Gynecology*, 132, 495–500.

Lederman R P, Lederman R, Work B A and McCann D S (1979), Relationship of psychological factors in pregnancy to progress in labour, *Nursing Research*, 28, 94–6.

Levin J S and DeFrank R S (1988), Maternal stress and pregnancy outcomes: a review of the psychological literature, *Review of Psychosomatic Obstetrics and Gynaecology*, 9, 3–16.

Lewis E (1982), Attendance for antenatal care, *British Medical Journal*, 284, 788.

Ley P (1977), Psychological studies of doctor–patient communication. In S Rachmann (Ed.) *Contributions to Medical Psychology*, Vol 1, Oxford: Pergamon.

Ley P (1982), Giving information to patients. In J R Eiser (Ed.) *Social Psychology and Behavioral Medicine*, Chichester: Wiley.

Ley P (1988), *Communicating with Patients*, London: Chapman & Hall.

Ley P, Bradshaw P W, Kincey J and Atherton S T (1976a), Increasing patients' satisfaction with communication, *British Journal of Sociology and Clinical Psychology*, 15, 217–20.

Ley P and Spelman M (1967), *Communicating with the Patient*, London: Staples Press.

Ley P, Whitworth M A, Skilbeck C E, Woodward R, Pinsent R, Pike L A, Clarkson M E and Clark P B (1976b), Improving doctor–patient communications in general practice, *Journal of the Royal College of General Practitioners*, 26, 720–4.

Little R (1977), Moderate alcohol use during pregnancy and decreased infant birth weight, *American Journal of Public Health*, 67, 1154–6.

Little R E, Asker R L, Sampson P D and Renwick J H (1986), Fetal growth and moderate drinking in early pregnancy, *American Journal of Epidemiology*, 123, 270–8.

Lloyd B W (1984), Outcome of very-low-birthweight babies from Wolverhampton, *Lancet*, September 29, 739–41.

Lowe R and Frey J (1983), Predicting Lamaze childbirth intentions and outcomes: an extension of the Theory of Reasoned Action to a joint outcome, *Basic and Applied Social Psychology*, 4, 353–72.

Lucas A, Morley R, Cole T J, Bamford M F, Boon A, Crowle P, Dossetor J F B and Pearce R (1988), Maternal fitness and viability of preterm infants, *British Medical Journal*, 296, 1495–7.

Lucas P and Lucas A (1980), Down's syndrome: telling the parents, *British Journal of Mental Subnormality*, 26, 21–31.

Lunenfield E, Rosenthal J, Larholt K M and Insler V (1984), Childbirth experience – psychological, cultural and medical associations, *Journal of Psychosomatic Obstetrics and Gynaecology*, 3, 165–71.

MacArthur C, Newton J R and Knox E G (1987), Effect of anti-smoking health education on infant size at birth: a randomized controlled trial, *British Journal of Obstetrics and Gynaecology*, 94, 295–300.

Macfarlane A and Mugford M (1984), *Birth Counts: Statistics of Pregnancy and Childbirth*. National Perinatal Epidemiological Unit (in collaboration with OPCS). London: HMSO.

Manstead A S R, Proffitt C and Smart J L (1983), Predicting and understanding mothers' infant-feeding intentions and behaviour: testing the theory of reasoned action, *Journal of Personality and Social Psychology*, 44, 657–71.

Marlow N, D'Souza S W and Chiswick M L (1987), Neurodevelopmental outcome in babies weighing less than 2001g at birth, *British Medical Journal*, 294, 1582–6.

Martin J and Roberts C (1984), *Women and Employment*, London: OPCS.

Martin T R and Bracken M S (1986), Association of low birth weight with passive smoke exposure in pregnancy, *American Journal of Epidemiology*, 124, 633–42.

Maternity Services Advisory Committee (1982), *Maternity Care in Action*. Part I: *Antenatal Care. First Report of the Maternity Services Advisory Committee*, London: HMSO.

McDonald R L, (1968), The role of emotional factors in obstetric complications: A review, *Psychosomatic Medicine*, 30, 222–36.

McIntosh J (1989), Models of childbirth and social class: a study of 80 working-class primigravidae. In S Robinson and A M Thomson (Eds.), *Midwives, Research and Childbirth*, Vol. I, London: Chapman & Hall, 189–214.

McKinlay J B (1970), The new late comers for antenatal care, *British Journal of Preventive Social Medicine*, 24, 52–7.

McKinlay J B (1973), Social networks, lay consultation and help-seeking behaviour, *Social Forces*, 51, 275–92.

McKinlay J B and McKinlay S M (1979), The influence of a pre-marital conception and various obstetric complications on subsequent prenatal health behaviour, *Journal of Epidemiology and Community Health*, 33, 84–90.

Midgley J M and MacRae A W (1971), Audio-visual media in general practice, *Journal of the Royal College of General Practitioners*, 21, 346–51.

Molfese V J, Bricker M C, Manion L G, Beadnell B, Yaple K and Moires K A (1987), Anxiety, depression and stress in pregnancy: a multivariate model of intra-partum risks and pregnancy outcomes, *Journal of Psychosomatic Obstetrics and Gynaecology*, 7, 77–92.

Murphy J F, Daulncey M, Newcombe R, Garcia J and Elbourne D (1984), Employment in pregnancy: prevalence, maternal characteristics, perinatal outcome, *Lancet*, 26 May, 1163–6.

National Association for Mental Health (1971): Carr E F and Oppé T E (Eds.), The birth of an abnormal child: telling the parents, *Lancet*, 2, 1075–7.

Nelson K B and Ellenberg J H (1986), Antecedents of cerebral palsy:

multivariate analysis of risk, *New England Journal of Medicine*, 315, 81–6.

Nelson M (1983), Working-class women, middle-class women and models of childbirth, *Social Problems*, 30, 284–97.

Nelson M K (1982), The effect of childbirth preparation on women of different social classes, *Journal of Health and Social Behaviour*, 23, 339–52.

Nettelbladt P, Fagerstom C and Uddenberg N (1976), The significance of reported childbirth pain, *Journal of Psychosomatic Research*, 20, 215–21.

Newton R W and Hunt L P (1984), Psychosocial stress in pregnancy and its relation to low birthweight, *British Medical Journal*, 288, 1191–4.

Newton R W, Webster P A, Binu P S, Maskrey N and Phillips A B (1979), Psychosocial stress in pregnancy and its relation to the onset of premature labour, *British Medical Journal*, 2, 411–13.

Norbeck J S and Tilden V P (1983), Life stress, social support and emotional disequilibrium in complications of pregnancy: a prospective multivariate study, *Journal of Health and Social Behaviour*, 24, 30–46.

Norr K L, Block C R, Charles A, Meyering S and Meyers E (1977), Explaining pain and enjoyment in childbirth, *Journal of Health and Social Behaviour*, 18, 260–75.

Nuckolls K B, Cassel J and Kaplan B H (1972), Psychosocial assets, life crisis and the prognosis of pregnancy, *American Journal of Epidemiology*, 95, 431–41.

O'Brien M and Smith C (1981), Women's views and experiences of antenatal care, *The Practitioner*, 225, 123–5.

O'Hara M W (1986), Social support, life-events and depression during pregnancy and the puerperium, *Archives of General Psychiatry*, 43, 569–73.

O'Reilly P (1988), Methodological issues in social support and social network research, *Social Science and Medicine*, 26, 863–73.

Oakley A (1974), *The Sociology of Housework*, London: Martin Robertson.

Oakley A (1977), *From Here to Maternity*, Harmondsworth: Penguin.

Oakley A (1980), *Women Confined*, Oxford: Martin Robertson.

Oakley A (1984), The effect of the mother's work on the infant. In G Chamberlain (Ed.) *Pregnant Women at Work*. London: Royal Society of Medicine, Macmillan.

Oakley A (1985), Social support in pregnancy: the 'soft' way to increase birthweight?, *Social Science and Medicine*, 21, 1259–68.

Oakley A (1989), Smoking in pregnancy: smokescreen or risk factor? Towards a materialist analysis, *Sociology of Health and Illness*, 11, 311–35.

Oakley A, MacFarlane A and Chalmers I (1982), Social class, stress and reproduction. In A R Rees and H J Purcell (Eds.) *Disease and the Environment*, Chichester: Wiley.

Oakley A and Rajan L (1991), Social class and social support: the same or different?, *Sociology*, 25, 31–59.

Oakley A, Rajan L and Grant A (1990), Social support and pregnancy outcome, *British Journal of Obstetrics and Gynaecology*, 97, 155–62.

Obayuwana A C, Carter A L and Barnett R M (1984), Psychosocial distress and pregnancy outcome: a three year prospective study, *Journal of Psychosomatic Obstetrical Gynaecology*, 3, 173–83.

Olshansky S (1962), Parent response to having a mentally defective child, *Social Casework*, 43, 190–3.

OPCS: Office of Population Censuses and Surveys (1988) *Hospital In-patient Enquiry Maternity Tables 1982–1985*, Series MB4, No 28, London: HMSO.

OPCS: Office of Population Censuses and Surveys (1989), *Women's Experience of Maternity Care – A Postal Survey Manual*, London: HMSO.

OPCS: Office of Population Censuses and Surveys (1990), *Standard Occupational Classification*, London: HMSO.

OPCS: Office of Population Censuses and Surveys (1991a), *General Household Survey: Cigarette Smoking 1972 to 1990*, Monitor, SS 91/3. London: OPCS.

OPCS: Office of Population Censuses and Surveys (1991b), *General Household Survey 1989*, London: OPCS.

Ounsted M, Moar V A and Scott A (1985), Risk factors associated with small-for-dates and large-for-dates pregnancies, *British Journal of Obstetrics and Gynaecology*, 92, 226–32.

Pagel M D, Smilkstein G, Regen H and Montano D (1990), Psychosocial influences on new born outcomes: a controlled prospective study, *Social Science and Medicine*, 30, 597–604.

Parker G and Barnett B (1987), A test of the social support hypothesis, *British Journal of Psychiatry*, 150, 72–7.

Pearlin L and Schooler C (1978), The structure of coping, *Journal of Health and Social Behaviour*, 19, 2–21.

Peters T J, Golding J, Butler N R, Fryer J E, Lawrence C J and Chamberlain E V P (1983), Plus ça change: predictors of birthweight in two national studies, *British Journal of Obstetrics and Gynaecology*, 90, 1040–5.

Peters T J, Adelstein P, Golding J and Butler N R (1984), The effects of work in pregnancy: short- and long-term associations. In G Chamberlain (Ed.) *Pregnant Women at Work*, London: Royal Society of Medicine/Macmillan.

Pickering R M (1987a), Maternal characteristics and the distribution of birthweight standardized for gestational age, *Journal of Biosocial Science*, 19, 17–26.

Pickering R M (1987b), Relative risks of low birthweight in Scotland 1980–2, *Journal of Epidemiology and Community Health*, 41, 133–9.

Pill R and Stott N C H (1982), Concepts of illness causation and responsibility: some preliminary data from a sample of working class mothers, *Social Science and Medicine*, 16, 43–52.

Pill R and Stott N C H (1985), Choice or chance: further evidence on ideas of illness and responsibility for health, *Social Science and Medicine*, 20, 981–91.

Pill R and Stott N C H (1987), Development of a measure of potential health behaviour: a salience of lifestyle index, *Social Science and Medicine*, 24, 125–34.

Pueschel S M and Murphy A (1976), Assessment of counselling practices at the birth of a child with Down's syndrome, *American Journal of Mental Deficiency*, 81, 325–30.

Pugh G and Russell P (1977), *Shared Care: Support Services for Families with Handicapped Children*, London: National Children's Bureau.

Quine L and Pahl J (1986), First diagnosis of severe mental handicap: characteristics of unsatisfactory encounters between doctors and parents, *Social Science and Medicine*, 22, 53–62.

Quine L and Pahl J (1987), First diagnosis of severe mental handicap: a study of parental reactions, *Developmental Medicine and Child Neurology*, 29, 232–42.

Quine L and Rutter D R (1993), Breaking the news of severe mental and physical disabilities: a study of doctor–parent communication, *Journal of Child Psychology and Psychiatry*, in press.

Quine L, Rutter D R and Gowen S (1993), Women's satisfaction with the quality of the birth experience: a prospective study of social and psychological predictors, *Journal of Infant and Reproductive Psychology*, in press.

Reading A E, Campbell S, Cox D M and Sledmere C M (1982), Health beliefs and health care behaviour in pregnancy, *Psychological Medicine*, 379–83.

Reid M E and McIlwaine G M (1980), Consumer opinion of a hospital antenatal clinic, *Social Science and Medicine*, 14, 363–68.

Ringrose C A (1972), Psychopathology of toxaemia of pregnancy. In J Howells (Ed.) *Modern Perspectives in Psycho-obstetrics*. Edinburgh: Oliver and Boyd, 283–91.

Robson J, Boomla K and Savage W (1986), Reducing delay in booking for antenatal care, *Journal of the Royal College of General Practitioners*, 36, 274–5.

Rosengren W R (1961), Some social psychological aspects of delivery room difficulties, *Journal of Nervous and Mental Disease*, 132, 515–21.

Roter D L (1977), Patient participation in the patient-provided interaction: the effects of patient question-asking on the quality of interaction satisfaction and compliance, *Health Education Monographs*, 5, 281–315.

Rubin D H, Krasilnikoff P A, Leventhal J M, Weile B and Berget A (1986), Effect of passive smoking on birth-weight, *Lancet*, August 23, 415–17.

Rush D (1982), Effects of change in protein and calorie intake during pregnancy on the growth of the human fetus. In M Enkin and I Chalmers (Eds.) *Effectiveness and Satisfaction in Antenatal Care*, London: Heinemann.

Russell M and Skinner J (1988), Early measures of maternal alcohol misuse as predictors of adverse pregnancy outcomes, *Alcoholism: Clinical and Experimental Research*, 12, 824–30.

Rutter D R (1980), A programme of interview training for medical students. In W T Singleton, P Spurgeon and R B Stammers (Eds.) *The Analysis of Social Skill*, New York: Plenum, 291–303.

Rutter D R and Maguire P (1976), Training medical students to communicate: the development and evaluation of an interviewing model and training procedure. In A E Bennett (Ed.) *Communication Between Doctors and Patients*, London: Oxford University Press, 47–74.

Rutter D R, Quine L and Hayward R (1988), Satisfaction with maternity care: psychosocial factors in pregnancy outcome, *Journal of Reproductive and Infant Psychology*, 6, 261–9.

Rutter M, Tizard J and Whitmore K (1970), *Education, Health and Behaviour*, London: Longman.

Sanjose S, Ramon E and Beral V (1991), Low birthweight and preterm delivery, Scotland, 1981–84: effect of parents' occupation, *Lancet*, 338, 428–31.

Saurel-Cubizolles M J, Kaminski M, Llado-Arkhipoff J, Du Mazaubrun C, Estryn-Behar M, Berthier C, Mouchet M and Kelfa C (1985), Pregnancy and its outcome among hospital personnel according to occupation and working conditions, *Journal of Epidemiology and Community Health*, 39, 129–34.

Schofield L, Wheeler E and Stewart J (1987), The diets of pregnant and post-pregnant women in different social groups in London and Edinburgh: energy, protein, fat and fibre, *British Journal of Nutrition*, 58, 369–81.

Scott-Samuel A (1980), Why don't they want our health services?, *Lancet*, 23 February, 412.

Sexton M and Habel J R (1984), A clinical trial of change in maternal smoking and its effects on birthweight, *Journal of the American Medical Association*, 251, 911–25.

Simpson H and Walker G (1980), When do pregnant women attend for antenatal care?, *British Medical Journal*, 12 July, 104–7.

Simpson R J and Smith N G (1986), Maternal smoking and low birthweight: implications for antenatal care, *Journal of Epidemiology and Community Health*, 140, 223–7.

Simpson W J (1957), A preliminary report of cigarette smoking and incidence of prematurity, *American Journal of Obstetrics and Gynecology*, 73, 808.

Skeoch C, Rosenberg K, Turner T, Skeoch H and McIlwaine G (1987), Very low birthweight survivors: illness and readmission to hospital in the first 15 months of life, *British Medical Journal*, 295, 579–80.

Smith B and Phillips C J (1978), Identification of severe handicap, *Child: Care, Health and Development*, 4, 195–203.

Solnit A J and Stark H M (1961), Mourning the birth of a defective child, *The Psychoanalytic Study of the Child*, 16, 523–37.

Sosa R, Kennell J, Klaus M, Robertson S and Urrutia J (1980), The effect of a supportive companion on perinatal problems, length of labor and mother–infant interaction, *The New England Journal of Medicine*, 303, 597–600.

Springer A and Steele M W (1980), Effects of physicians' early parental counselling on rearing Down's syndrome children, *American Journal of Mental Deficiency*, 85, 1–5.

Stanley F J and English D R (1986), Prevalence of and risk factors for cerebral palsy in a total population cohort of low-birthweight (< 2000g) infants, *Developmental Medicine and Child Neurology*, 28, 559–68.

Stein Z A, Susser M, Saeneger G and Marolla F (1975), *Famine and Human Development: The Dutch Hunger Winter of 1944–45*, New York: Oxford University Press.

Stein Z A, Susser M W and Hatch M C (1986), Working during pregnancy: physical and psychosocial strain, *Occupational Medicine: State of the Art Reviews*, 1, 405–9.

Stevens D P, Staff R N and MacKay C R (1977), What happens when hospitalized patients see their records?, *Annals of International Medicine*, 86, 474–7.

Stewart M (1984), What is a successful doctor–patient interview? A study of interactions and outcomes, *Social Science and Medicine*, 19, 167–75.

Sulaiman N D du V, Florey C, Taylor D J and Ogston S A (1988), Alcohol consumption in Dundee primigravidas and its effects on outcome of pregnancy, *British Medical Journal*, 296, 1500–3.

Svarstad B and Lipton H L (1977), Informing parents about mental retardation: a study of professional communication and parent acceptance, *Social Science and Medicine*, 11, 645–51.

Taylor A (1986), Maternity services: the consumer's view, *Journal of the Royal College of General Practitioners*, 36, 157–60.

Thoits P A (1982), Conceptual methodological and theoretical views in studying social support as a buffer against life stress, *Journal of Health and Social Behaviour*, 23, 145–59.

UK Royal College of Physicians (1983), *Health or Smoking?* London: Pitman.

UK Royal College of Psychiatrists (1982), Alcohol and alcoholism, *Bulletin of the Royal College of Psychiatrists*, 6, 69.

US Surgeon General (1980), *The Health Consequences of Smoking for Women*, Washington DC: US Department of Health and Human Services.

US Surgeon General (1981), Surgeon General's advice on alcohol and pregnancy, *FDA Drug Bulletin*, 11, 9–10.

Wallston B S and Wallston K A (1978a), Locus of control and health: a review of the literature, *Health Education Monographs*, 6, 107–17.

Wallston K A and Wallston B S (1978b), Development of the multidimensional health locus of control (MHLC) scale, *Health Education Monographs*, 6, 160–70.

Wallston K A and Wallston B S (1981), Health locus of control scales. In H M Lefcourt (Ed.) *Research with the Locus of Control Constant.* Vol.1: *Assessment Methods*, New York: Academic Press.

Waterson E J and Murray-Lyon I M (1990), Preventing alcohol related birth damage: a review, *Social Science and Medicine*, 30, 349–64.

Weiner L, Rosett H L, Edelkin C, Alpert J and Zuckerman B (1983), Alcohol consumption by pregnant women, *Obstetrical Gynaecology*, 61, 6–12.

Westbrook M T (1979), Socio-economic differences in coping with childbearing, *American Journal of Community Psychology*, 7, 397–411.

Whitehead A (1987), *The Health Divide: Inequalities in Health in the 1980's*, London: Health Education Council.

Wolkind S and Zajicek E (Eds.) (1981), *Pregnancy: A Psychosocial and Social Study*, London: Academic Press.

Wright J T, Barrison I G, Lewis I G, MacRae K D, Waterson E J, Toplis P J, Gordon M G, Morris N F and Murray-Lyon M L (1983), Alcohol consumption, pregnancy and low birthweight, *Lancet*, 26 March, 663–5.

Yang R, Zweig A, Ponthitt T and Federman E (1976), Successive relationships between maternal attitudes during pregnancy, analgesic medication during labour and delivery and newborn behaviour, *Developmental Psychology*, 12, 6–14.

Yerushalmy J (1971), The relationship of parents' cigarette smoking to outcome of pregnancy – implications of the problem of inferring causation from observed associations, *American Journal of Epidemiology*, 93, 443–56.

Young G (1987), Are isolated maternity units run by general practitioners dangerous?, *British Medical Journal*, 294, 744–6.

Zajicek E (1981), The experience of being pregnant. In S Wolkind and E Zajicek (Eds.) *Pregnancy: A Psycho-social and Social Study*. London: Academic Press.

Chapter 3

Breast Cancer Screening

One in twelve women in the United Kingdom develops breast cancer. Almost 15,000 die of it each year, more than from any other form of cancer, and the disease now accounts among women for one in five cancer deaths and one in twenty deaths overall. The figures have risen steadily for many years and are the worst in Western Europe and possibly the world. What causes the disease, however, and how to prevent it are not yet understood, but it is well established that early detection offers the most hopeful prognosis. The main purpose of this chapter is to identify the principal social inputs for mortality, incidence and survival, to trace the paths of mediation and to present our own research on social psychological factors in screening.

There are four sections. The first presents the published epidemiological statistics, and it emerges that age, social class, marriage and motherhood are the leading social inputs. The most important mediator between inputs and outcomes is early diagnosis – but the only way at present to achieve early diagnosis over the population as a whole is to ensure that women attend for regular X-ray mammography, perhaps in conjunction with self-examination. The key issue for social psychological research is who does and does not attend for screening, and why. The literature on screening takes up the second section of the chapter, first the medical literature on effectiveness, and then the psychological and social psychological literature on attendance and acceptability. In the third section we report our own programme of research, from our early work on attitudes and breast self-examination to our current research into X-ray mammography and 'consumer satisfaction' with services. The final section discusses the implications of our findings for theory, policy and practice.

The epidemiology of breast cancer

Mortality

In the most recent year for which published statistics are available, 1990, more than 13,600 women died of breast cancer in England and Wales (Figure 3.1). The figure has risen steadily since the mid-1970s, and the disease now kills more women than any other form of cancer – almost 30 per cent more than lung cancer, for example, and over 750 per cent more than cervical cancer. England and Wales have the highest rate in the European Community and one of the highest in the world. The figures are strongly age-related, but, even though the majority of deaths occur in older age, more women die from breast cancer in the age group 35–54 than from any other single cause.

One of the questions epidemiologists are now asking is whether mortality may be associated with social inputs. In this country, as we saw in Chapter 1, one of the major sources of data is the OPCS Longitudinal Study, a long-term national examination of demographic and health trends. From the 1971 Census, a 1 per cent random sample of the population was taken, and from official returns the 250,000 males and 250,000 females who make up the sample are being followed until they die. An enormous amount of information has already been collected, all of it unobtrusively and unknown to the subjects, and a variety of important issues which would otherwise be quite impossible to approach are gradually being resolved.

One of the items of information collected routinely in the Longitudinal Study is cancer diagnoses, since every case of cancer is now registered centrally under the National Cancer Registration Scheme introduced in England and Wales in 1971. By cross-referencing cancer registrations with all its other information, the Longitudinal Study has already been able to point to two important social inputs in breast cancer mortality. First, mortality

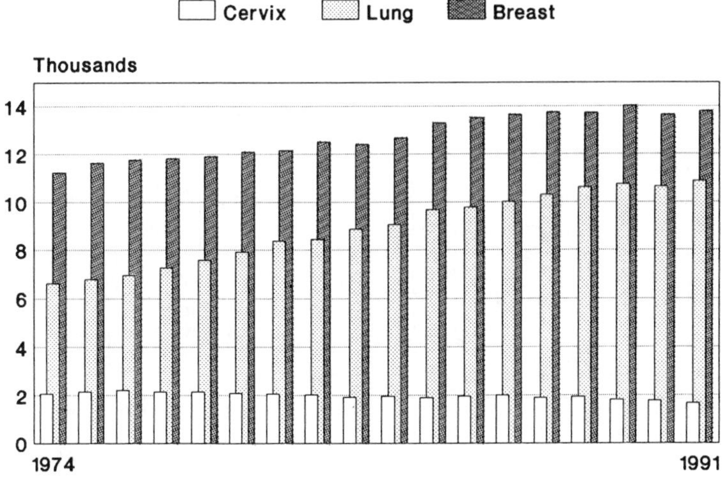

Figure 3.1 Cancer deaths among women. Source: OPCS Series DH2, statistics are for England and Wales

is lowest in women with non-manual occupations – as it is for cervical cancer – and the comparison between non-manual and manual reaches statistical significance. Second, mortality is highest in women who have not had children while, among those who have, it is lowest in those who first gave birth in their twenties. The large sample size, the prospective nature of the design, and the routine and unobtrusive way the data are collected make the findings particularly reliable.

Incidence

From the mid-1970s, over 20,000 new cases of breast cancer have been diagnosed each year in England and Wales (Figure 3.2). As with mortality, the most interesting question from our point of view is whether there is any association with social inputs, and again social class and motherhood have received the most attention. The principal facts, according to data from national

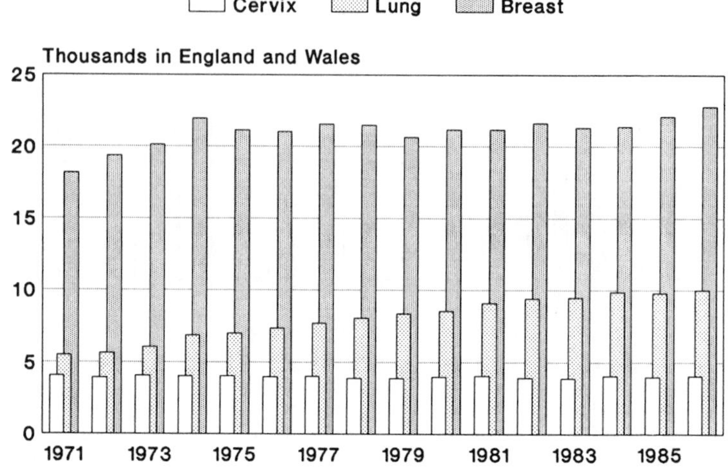

Figure 3.2 Cancer incidence among women. Source: OPCS Series MB1. Cancer statistics – registrations

cancer registrations and from the OPCS Longitudinal Study, are that women in Classes I and II have a raised incidence compared with those in the remaining classes, and that women who have had two or more children are the least at risk. Why motherhood should be protective is unclear, though there is evidence that lactation may be an important variable, while breastfeeding appears not to be (Doll and Peto, 1986). The older the woman when her first child is born, the greater her subsequent risk – something which may help to explain the findings for social class since women in Classes I and II have their children later on average than those in other classes.

Survival

The central questions about survival are how many people survive cancer once they have contracted it, and for how long. The first statistic is crude survival rate. Again we rely on the Longitudinal Study for our findings, and it emerges that five years after diagnosis 50 per cent of women with breast cancer are still alive: the figure is the same for cervical cancer, against 5 per cent for lung cancer and 36 per cent for cancer overall (Figure 3.3).[1] An alternative way of expressing the data is to present median survival time – that is, the number of years after diagnosis at which 50 per cent of patients are still alive. The figures are 5 years for breast cancer, 5 years 2 months for cervical cancer, and 4 months for lung cancer. The only input variable to have received significant attention is social class, but median survival time appears to be relatively unaffected by it.

Causes, prevention and treatment

What causes breast cancer and how to prevent it are unknown. A variety of possible causal factors has been suggested from genetic predisposition to exogenous factors such as diet (especially fat), oral contraceptives and oestrogen in hormone replacement therapy – but the evidence is not yet conclusive (Doll and Peto, 1986). Without detailed knowledge of causal mechanisms, there is little hope of prevention, and all that remains is to treat the disease when it is detected. Advances in surgery, radiotherapy, chemotherapy and hormone therapy have led to small increases in survival time following treatment, but the most important determinant of how long a patient survives is not the type of treatment but how early the disease is detected, so that treatment of whatever sort can begin. Many patients first present to their doctor so late that their tumour is easily palpable and is probably so advanced that treatment will fail. The only way to reduce mortality substantially is to detect the disease before the patient notices symptoms – and the only feasible way to do that at present is through mass population screening by X-ray mammography.

Breast cancer starts in the milk-producing cells of the breast

1. Data from the National Cancer Registration Scheme for the entire population of England and Wales reveal five-year survival figures of 49 per cent for breast cancer, 48 per cent for cervical cancer, 5 per cent for lung cancer and 35 per cent for cancer overall – indicating that the Longitudinal Study's 1 per cent sample is impressively representative.

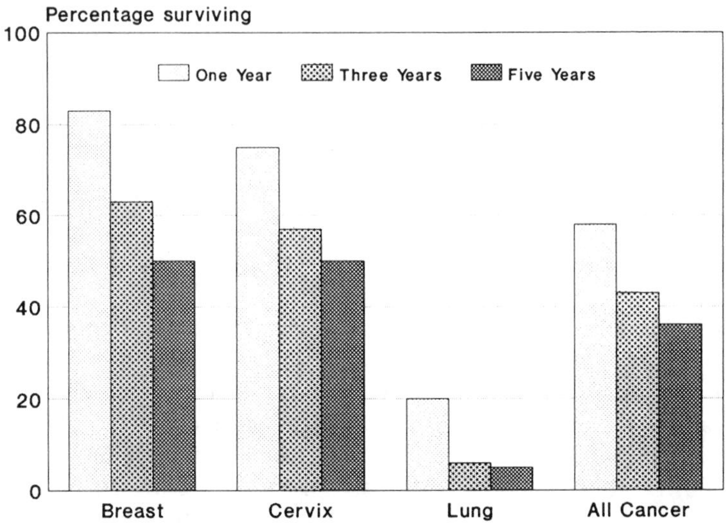

Figure 3.3 Cancer crude survival rates, 1971–83. Source: OPCS Longitudinal Study

and in the cells lining the milk ducts. In the 'pre-invasive' stage, malignant cells are confined to the duct system. In the invasive phase, the cancer attacks the surrounding tissues and has the potential to spread to local lymph nodes and to distant sites, such as bones, the liver and the brain. The rate of growth of the cancer cells varies from woman to woman, and the development of metastases may not occur for many years. The object of screening is to detect the disorder while it is confined to the breast, if possible while it is still pre-invasive. As many as 80 per cent of cancers that are too small to be detected by clinical examination – probably less than 1 cm in diameter – are nevertheless invasive and may have spread to local lymph nodes and even more distant sites. At present, X-ray mammography is the only technique for detecting such small abnormalities in the mass population.

Social inputs and mediators: the role of screening

X-ray mammography and its effectiveness

Mammography is normally conducted by a radiographer, using X-ray equipment specially designed for the one specific purpose. The woman stands, and is positioned so that the entire breast can be 'photographed' in one shot, normally above, to the side, through the middle. A similar mammogram is then made of the other breast. The developed films are read in batches, typically by a radiologist, but sometimes by another doctor or health professional. The reading is done by eye, and the decision as to whether there is or is not evidence of cancer is generally taken in a matter of seconds by just the one person. If there is doubt, a second pair of mammograms will probably be taken but, if whoever reads the film sees evidence of cancer, the woman will be recalled for further investigation.

Any form of screening sorts cases into 'test positives' and 'test negatives'. By the very nature of detection tests, some of the test positives will in fact be negatives (that is, they are *false* positives and do not have the disease), and some of the test negatives will be positives (false negatives who do have the disease). In any screening test, the criterion for selection is controlled by the tester, and can be moved up or down so that either false positives or false negatives are minimized. The difficulty, of course, is that the two are inversely related, so that reducing false negatives will mean increasing false positives, and vice versa.

The number of true positives detected by screening as a proportion of all the women in the sample who actually have cancer is known as the sensitivity of the test (Figure 3.4). The corresponding index for negatives – the number of true negatives detected as a proportion of all the women in the sample without cancer – is the specificity of the test. The goal is to have both sensitivity and specificity as high as possible. Current figures from the major British centres average more than 90 per cent for sensitivity and a little higher for specificity. In other words, 5–10 per cent of breast cancers are missed and 5–10 per cent of women who do not have cancer are wrongly defined as positive cases. 'Missed' cancers are those that are found within twelve months of the screen and, since some of them will not have started until

		True Diagnosis	
		Breast Cancer Present	Breast Cancer Absent
Test result	Positive	True Positive (a)	False positive (c)
	Negative	False negative (b)	True negative (d)

Sensitivity is the number of true positives as a proportion of all those with breast cancer present

i.e. $\frac{(a)}{(a)+(b)}$

Specificity is the number of true negatives as a proportion of all those with breast cancer absent

i.e. $\frac{(d)}{(c)+(d)}$

Figure 3.4 Sensitivity and specificity of screening test for breast cancer

after the screen, the number of genuinely missed cancers is probably rather lower than the figures for sensitivity suggest.

The question for research has been to investigate systematically how effective X-ray mammography is, and the dependent measure used most frequently has been lives saved. Three main approaches have developed, and the first has been to set up case-control studies. A population of women, typically 20,000–30,000, is invited to be screened at regular intervals, and all deaths from breast cancer are logged from clinical records or death certificates. Each woman who dies of breast cancer is then matched retrospectively with women who are still alive. Normally, up to five 'controls' will be examined for each 'case', and matching will be based on age, since age is a strong predictor of death. The question is simply what proportion of cases and what proportion of controls will be found to have attended for screening.

The three leading case-control studies are all from Europe – Nijmegen, Utrecht and Florence – and all report a marked association between screening and reduced mortality. In Nijmegen (Verbeek *et al.*, 1984), 23,000 women aged 35–65 were invited for a first screen in 1975, and then again on three more occasions at two-yearly intervals. Additional women were included in the subsequent rounds, giving a final total of over 30,000. By the end of 1981, six years after screening began, 46 women had died of breast cancer – of whom 26 had been screened at least once, and 20 had not. Of the 130 controls who were matched with screened cases, 100 had been screened; of the 100 matched with unscreened cases, 62 had been screened. The odds ratio estimated from the figures was 0.48 which, when translated into lives saved, means that 52 per cent of screened women who 'ought' to have died had not. Screening, according to the logic of case-control designs, was what had saved them. In Utrecht (Collette *et al.*, 1984), where screening was repeated 12, 18 and 24 months after the first occasion, the saving was estimated at 70 per cent after 8 years in women aged 50–64 at first invitation. In Florence (Palli *et al.*, 1989), the estimate was 50 per cent for women over 50 who had been screened within 30 months of monitoring. There was no noticeable advantage to women under 50.

Though the apparent effect of screening is dramatic in case-control studies, there is a serious methodological worry: women who choose to be screened may be the least at risk of breast cancer (see, for example, the report by the UK Trial of Early Detection of Breast Cancer group, 1988). If that were so, the saving in mortality might be less attributable to screening than to the characteristics of the woman or her circumstances which led her to be screened – something that no amount of retrospective matching can hope to overcome. Case-control studies can never be conclusive, therefore, and what is needed is randomized prospective trials in which women are assigned at random to be invited for screening or not invited for screening. Between case-control studies and prospective randomized trials there is, however, an intermediate approach, which might be called the quasi-random trial, in which all women in one geographical area are invited for screening while those in another are not. The two groups are then compared for mortality in subsequent years. What is lost in comparison with a full randomized design is scientific rigour, for the two areas may differ in some uncontrolled way that happens to be associated with outcome; what is gained is the comparative ease of conducting the study.

The most noticeable example of a quasi-random study is the United Kingdom Trial of Early Detection of Breast Cancer (UK TEDBC group, 1988). Eight centres took part in the study, and in two of them (Edinburgh and Guildford) women were offered X-ray mammography, in two (Huddersfield and Nottingham) they were offered classes in self-examination, and in the remaining four (Dundee, Oxford, Southmead, Stoke) women were identified but not contacted and so had available to them only the routine services that existed already. The experimental period was seven years and, in the mammography group, X-ray mammography and clinical examination were offered in years 1, 3, 5 and 7, with clinical examination alone in years 2, 4 and 6. The women were all aged 45–64 at entry and there were over 45,000 in the mammography group, over 60,000 in the self-examination group and almost 130,000 in the control group. The trial began in 1979, all the women to be included had started by 1981, and mortality was first assessed at the end of 1986. The results showed a saving of 20 per cent mortality in the mammography group, and a slight excess mortality in the self-examination group, but neither figure reached statistical significance. The data might, of course, have shown a stronger pattern for older women, as in the case-control studies, but no breakdown by age was carried out. Attendance figures for the first screen, it should be noted, were 72 per cent for Guildford and 60 per cent for Edinburgh.

The authors of the papers on the UK TEDBC acknowledge that quasi-random trials are hard to interpret. The only satisfactory approach is the fully randomized prospective trial. From a defined population, women are selected at random to be invited for screening or not invited for screening, and the number of deaths from breast cancer in each of the two groups is logged as time passes. The confounding of geographical factors encountered in the quasi-random trial is thus avoided and the best possible estimate of the effects of screening is obtained.

There have been four major randomized controlled trials (Table 3.1), the first of them conducted by the Health Insurance Plan in New York, starting in 1963 (Shapiro, 1977; Habbema *et al.*, 1986). A total of 31,000 women were invited for screening, and a further 31,000 were not. All were aged 40–64 at entry, and mortality has so far been monitored for eighteen years. The estimated saving in mortality in the invited group up to the end of 1990 was 21 per cent, and the figure was the same for women aged 50 and over.

The second trial to be set up was the Malmo trial in 1976 (Andersson *et al.*, 1988; Andersson, 1989). There followed the Swedish Two Counties trial in 1977 (Tabar *et al.*, 1985; Tabar *et al.*, 1989; Fagerberg, 1989), and the Edinburgh trial in 1979, which was a randomized controlled addition to the UK TEDBC

Table 3.1 Randomized controlled trials of mammography to end of 1990

	Method[a]	Interval in years	Rounds	Age at entry	Initial acceptance	Follow-up in years	Mortality vs. control
HIP, New York 1963 →	M+P	1	4	40–64 50+	65%	18[b]	−21% −21%
Malmo Sweden 1976 →	M	1–2	5	45–69 56+	74%	11	−17% −27%
Two Counties, Sweden 1977 →	M	2–3	3	40–74 50+	89%	8	−30% −34%
Edinburgh 1979 →	M+P	2	4	45–64 50+	61%	7	−16% −20%

Adapted from Vessey (1991).
Number invited for screening ranges from 21,000 (Malmo) to 77,000 (Two Counties).
[a] M = Mammography; P = Palpation.
[b] Cases diagnosed within five years of randomization.

(Samuel *et al.*, 1978; Roberts, 1989; Roberts *et al.*, 1990). In each case, the design was essentially the same as in New York, but follow-up has necessarily been shorter because of the later start: eleven years in Malmo, eight years in the Swedish Two Counties, and seven years in Edinburgh. In Malmo, the overall saving in the invited group was 17 per cent, in the Swedish Two Counties 30 per cent, and in Edinburgh 16 per cent. In all three studies, there was a clear benefit to older women: 27 per cent in Malmo (55+), 34 per cent in the Swedish Two Counties (50+), and 20 per cent in Edinburgh (50+). Not all the figures reached statistical significance, but the trend in all four studies was clear, at least for older women. Attendance rates for first screen were 65 per cent in New York, 74 per cent in Malmo, 89 per cent in the Swedish Two Counties and 61 per cent in Edinburgh. It should be noted that mortality figures for women in the 'invited for screening' groups include both attenders and non-attenders.

The results for attenders would no doubt be better than for non-attenders, but the difference has generally not been examined since the mass population result is what matters most in population screening. It is estimated from the Forrest programme in this country that, if 70 per cent of invited women accept their invitation, the reduction in mortality will be some 25 per cent, assuming that the programme continues to invite just women aged 50–64 (Vessey, 1991).

Reactions to the findings have been mixed, and the difficult issues they raise have led to a sometimes acrimonious debate between those who support the idea of national programmes of population screening and those who do not. The principal issues are these: screening may save 'a few' lives, but does it lead to an *overall* saving in mortality – that is, do people simply die of something else, at about the time they would have died of breast cancer? Does the financial cost of an effective service outweigh the benefits? Are there so many 'interval' cancers, those that develop between screens, that only a minority of cancers will be detected with, say, a three-yearly recall? Do false positives produce so much anxiety and psychological difficulty that the benefits of screening are outweighed? Is the same true of national publicity? Do X-rays produce physical damage, and does the same happen with biopsies and other examinations that a positive screen will make necessary? And what does knowing that she has cancer, perhaps in an advanced untreatable form, do to the woman psychologically and to her quality of life in whatever time she has left – might it be better not to know?

A discussion of the arguments is beyond the scope of the present book, but the interested reader is referred to Wright (1986), Miller (1988), Warren (1988), Skrabanek (1988), Reidy and Hoskins (1988) and Roberts (1989). Suffice to say that, in the United Kingdom, the issues were considered by a specialist Government committee, under Sir Patrick Forrest, which reported in 1986 that a national programme *should* be set up (Forrest, 1986). The report was accepted by the Government, and the programme began in 1988 and will run for an experimental period of three years. All women aged 50–64 are to be invited for mammography every three years, wherever in the United Kingdom they live. A central question, if the experiment is to be allowed to continue, will be how many women will accept their invitation. It is no surprise that Edinburgh, with the lowest saving of lives of the four randomized trials, had the lowest attendance rate at first screen (61 per cent), while the Swedish Two Counties, with the highest saving, had the highest attendance (89 per cent). If women do not attend, the experiment will fail. As to what it is that makes one woman attend but another not, we hope to provide answers in the second and third sections of the chapter.

Breast self-examination and its effectiveness

For most women, the main alternative to X-ray mammography is to examine their own breasts, perhaps with intermittent clinical examination by their family doctor. Self-examination was recognized as a screening technique long before mammography became available through national programmes, and many health districts and voluntary organizations in the United Kingdom provide classes to teach women the proper techniques. It is recommended that the woman examine her breasts once a month: she should check visually for changes in the skin or the size of the breasts, and for discharge, bleeding or unusually prominent veins; and she should feel systematically for lumps in and around the breasts and under the arms. Careful routines are prescribed, and the woman is advised to consult her doctor immediately if she suspects an abnormality of any sort.

As with X-ray mammography, the most important question to ask is whether self-examination saves lives, and again in principal there are three possible types of study: case-control studies, quasi-random studies and prospective randomized studies. In fact, though, there have been no studies of the third type, and our discussion will therefore be restricted to the first two. The most useful of the reports on case-control studies is by Hill *et al.* (1988). They identify twelve studies that had investigated women with breast cancer to find out whether they had practised self-examination before their illness had been detected. There were 8,118 cases in total, and Hill *et al.* combined the results of the studies statistically, using meta-analysis – a technique that allows a single estimate to be made of the effect of the variable in question, allowing for the statistical power and direction of results of each of the studies in turn. There were two main findings: significantly fewer of the women who had practised self-examination presented with tumours measuring 2 cm or more in diameter (56 per cent against 66 per cent); and significantly fewer had cancer in the lymph nodes (39 per cent against 50 per cent). The authors could not comment on mortality, since that was not under investigation in their particular study, but they did conclude that self-examination appeared to detect cancer at an earlier stage than no screening at all – and so, by implication, treatment would begin sooner. Note, however, that the analysis of tumour size took 2 cm diameter as its criterion – much bigger than the minimum size for X-ray mammography to detect, and probably already too advanced for successful intervention.

A further case-control study, not included by Hill *et al.*, was reported by Mant *et al.* (1987). They interviewed women newly diagnosed with breast cancer to find out if they had practised self-examination before their illness was discovered and, if so, whether they had been taught. Practising without teaching, it emerged, was no better than failing to practise at all. Women who practised and had been taught, however, had 'more favourable' tumours: 45 per cent had tumours 2 cm or less in diameter against 33 per cent of those who did not practise; 42 per cent had tumours at clinical stage 1 against 27 per cent; and in 50 per cent the cancer had not yet reached the axillary nodes, against 37 per cent. In other words, teaching had led women to detect tumours early, before they had begun to spread. Again, however, the question that remains is whether even earlier detection is necessary if mortality is to be reduced significantly.

The second type of study is the quasi-random trial, and there are only two large-scale examples, so far as we know. The first is the UK TEDBC, in which, it will be recalled, women in two of the four experimental districts were offered classes in self-examination while, in the other two, there was X-ray mammography. In the remaining four districts, nothing was offered, though existing routine services were available as normal. Whereas a reduction in mortality *had* been found for X-ray mammography, there was no reduction for self-examination – in fact, there was a slight, but non-significant, excess. The most telling part of the analysis, however, was the revelation that attendance rates for self-examination classes were 30 per cent in one district and 53 per cent in the other. Obvious questions are thus raised about the acceptability to women of self-examination classes, but nothing of any value can be said about mortality.

The other quasi-random study is a trial being conducted in Russia under the auspices of the World Health Organization (Tsechkovski *et al.*, 1986). The study is based on polyclinics in Saint Petersburg and factories in Moscow, and half the clinics and half the factories have been randomly chosen to be experimental sites, while the other half are control sites. Women who are registered with 'experimental' clinics or who work in 'experimental' factories are being offered group education in self-examination, and both incidence and mortality in the two cities are to be monitored for some years to come. No results are yet available.

Attendance rates and the acceptability of screening

Screening cannot succeed if women do not take part, and the findings in the previous section make it clear that many do not. The question is why. Is there evidence that social inputs are implicated, so that women of lower social class and education, for example, are less likely than middle-class, educated women to take up what is offered? Might attenders and non-attenders be different psychologically, perhaps in their views about preventive medicine, their beliefs about health and their attitudes to screening? And might social inputs and psychological measures be related, perhaps in the way that interests us especially, namely that social inputs are *mediated* by psychological and social psychological variables? For both X-ray mammography and self-examination there is a certain amount of published literature, though rather less than for the effectiveness of the techniques. The self-examination literature came first historically, since X-ray mammography arrived much later, and that is the order our own discussion will follow.

Breast self-examination

The most substantial work on breast self-examination has been conducted by our colleague Michael Calnan, and his collaborators. All Calnan's analyses have been based on data from the UK TEDBC, and the first asked two main questions: did women who attended self-examination classes differ in social inputs from those who turned down their invitation; and did they differ in their beliefs about health (Calnan and Moss, 1984). A total of 678 women who were to be invited to classes were interviewed shortly before their invitations arrived, and were then followed through to monitor whether they took up the invitation and to test how well they were carrying out self-examination.

Social inputs and health beliefs, it emerged, both distinguished between attenders and non-attenders: attenders were more likely than non-attenders to be from non-manual social classes, to have stayed at school beyond 16, and to be single or married (against widowed, divorced or separated); and they were more likely to see themselves as vulnerable to breast cancer and to be concerned about it. The other dimensions of the Health Belief Model did not separate the two groups, but attenders reported more encouragement and support from other people about going to classes than did non-attenders. They also reported 'better' personal health behaviours and greater use of preventive health services in general. When all the variables of interest were included in a discriminant analysis, the three strongest discriminators between attenders and non-attenders were found to be perceived vulnerability to breast cancer, use of preventive health services and personal health behaviours. As to how well the women were doing self-examination at Time 2 once the classes were over, the best predictors were frequency of doing self-examination at Time 1, social support, previous contact with self-examination education and self-examination technique at Time 1. The technique attenders were using was significantly better a year after classes than the technique of non-attenders at the equivalent time (Calnan, Chamberlain and Moss, 1983), and good technique was associated with a positive belief in the value of doing self-examination (Calnan, 1985).

A second line of questioning in Calnan's work has been whether women who do self-examination also do other preventive health behaviours, as the first findings had begun to suggest, and whether the social inputs that predicted one behaviour also predicted the others (Calnan and Rutter, 1986a). Doing self-examination, it emerged, was associated with wearing car seat belts (legislation to make it compulsory had not yet been passed), exercise, diet, regular visits to the dentist, cervical screening and breast screening; but there was no association with tooth brushing or smoking. Even the significant relationships were small, however, for the correlation coefficients ranged from 0.05 to 0.15, and so accounted for only 1 per cent or 2 per cent of the variance. As to social inputs, social class and education distinguished between 'doers' and 'non-doers' for every single behaviour except self-examination. Both inputs had predicted *attendance* at self-examination classes, but now, when the non-attenders and controls were added, there was no association with *performance*. The inputs that did predict were age and marriage: older women were less likely than younger women to do self-examination; and single, separated and divorced women were more likely to do it than those who were married or widowed.

The third and final line of questioning has concerned the detailed links between attitudes and behaviour. We knew already that beliefs predicted attendance and how well women were doing self-examination a year after the classes, but no attempt had been made to map the patterns of relationships over time. How much, for example, did beliefs at Time 1 influence behaviour at Time 2, irrespective of possible changes in beliefs between the two occasions; did beliefs at Time 2 matter at all to behaviour, or did women now behave by habit; and what effect did self-examination classes have on the links between beliefs and behaviour?

The analyses revealed three main findings (Calnan and Rutter, 1986b; Rutter and Calnan, 1987; Calnan and Rutter, 1988). First, the technique of self-examination used by the women improved from Time 1 to Time 2 in all three groups – attenders, non-attenders and controls. The improvement was greatest among attenders, and in the other groups was probably the result of publicity and perhaps the 'cueing' or 'triggering' effect of receiving and completing the Time 1 questionnaire. Second, beliefs did predict behaviour in all three groups at Time 2, but the proportion of variance explained was small, never more than 25 per cent in any of the three groups, and the perceived value of doing self-examination played a larger part than perceived vulnerability to breast cancer. Third, there was good evidence that habit was a significant factor, for technique at Time 1 was the best predictor for technique at Time 2 in all three groups. The pattern was complex, however: beliefs influenced behaviour at Time 2 directly, as well as indirectly through behaviour at Time 1; and the group for whom behaviour at Time 1 was least important was attenders. Classes thus helped women to improve their self-examination technique and so reduced the influence of Time 1 behaviour on Time 2 behaviour, but they also gave them a new underpinning for their behaviour by introducing new beliefs and information.

Apart from Calnan, the other main contributor has been Roberts, the Director of the Edinburgh Screening Centre, and once again social inputs emerge as important sources of variance. In the first of two studies, Roberts, French and Duffy (1984) interviewed a random sample of 810 women in Edinburgh to find out how much they knew about self-examination and how well they were doing it, if at all. Very few of the sample knew what to look for except lumps, and few were aware of any forms of treatment except mastectomy and radiotherapy. However, general knowledge about the breast and breast cancer was related to both age and social class: women aged 30–49 were more knowledgeable than those aged 18–29 or 50 and over; and, within each group, women from manual classes had lower scores than those from non-manual classes. Knowledge about how to do self-examination revealed a similar pattern, though women aged 50 or over were noticeably the least knowledgeable this time, in all social groups. Higher scores were often associated with personal experience of breast problems.

In the second study, Roberts went on from knowledge to attitudes (Leathar and Roberts, 1985). Again the subjects were women from Edinburgh, but this time the report was based on qualitative data from discussion groups. It was already clear from the Edinburgh randomized trial that 40 per cent of women turned down their invitation for X-ray mammography – attendance is generally much lower for self-examination classes, as we have seen (UK TEDBC group, 1988) – and the question was whether motivational and attitudinal factors might be responsible. The answer was that they were, and once again there were noticeable differences according to social inputs, especially age. The most important was that older women found self-examination distasteful, and this often led to the most cursory of examinations which could only fail. The authors concluded that health education that relies on mass media communication will succeed only if face-to-face communication, such as counselling, is incorporated with it.

X-ray mammography

There have been three main projects on X-ray mammography in this country, the first based on the UK TEDBC, the second conducted in Edinburgh, and the third conducted in Manchester. The UK TEDBC work was by Calnan and his colleagues (Calnan and Chamberlain, 1984; Calnan, 1984a, 1984b), and was concerned with how social inputs, beliefs and behaviour were related to attendance and non-attendance. Just one of the two mammography sites was investigated, Guildford, and the first thing to emerge was that, of all the social inputs studied, only age and marital status played a part – social class and school leaving age were not related to attendance for mammography though they had been related to attendance at self-examination classes. The effects for age and marital status were attributable to poor attendance in women over 60 and in those who were single or widowed. The main beliefs associated with attendance were high perceived vulnerability to breast cancer, faith that the disease could generally be cured and acceptance that the benefits of screening outweighed the costs. The main behaviours associated with attendance were previous use of screening services, notably cervical smears, dental checks and breast screening.

The second project, based in Edinburgh, began in a similar way, by examining the psychological characteristics of attenders and non-attenders (French *et al.*, 1982; Maclean *et al.*, 1984). While similar proportions of the two groups were aware of the benefits of early diagnosis and treatment, 58 per cent of non-attenders said one 'should not go looking for trouble' against 11 per cent of attenders, 79 per cent against 36 per cent were afraid of cancer being found, and 72 per cent against 13 per cent were anxious that their lives would be disrupted if it were. Demographic differences between the groups, and differences in the use of preventive health measures, were similar to those found in the UK TEDBC. The authors concluded that many women are afraid of screening and will not attend, thus reducing the chances that mass screening will succeed; but attempts to persuade them otherwise may not be justified since the evidence in favour of screening is as yet hardly decisive – not least, of course, precisely because attendance rates are so low.

In a later paper, the Edinburgh group went on to consider the perceived health status of attenders and non-attenders (Hunt, Alexander and Roberts, 1988). All women in Edinburgh invited for screening over a nine-month period were sent the Nottingham Health Profile questionnaire, which measures physical and psychological health (Hunt, McEwen and McKenna, 1986). The questionnaire was posted shortly after the invitation to screening had arrived, and almost 75 per cent responded of more than 2,200. Respondents were then broken down into four sub-groups: those who attended for screening; those who declined their invitation; those who failed to reply to the invitation; and those who accepted the invitation but then did not attend. The first three groups were found to be similar, and close to the population norm for their sex and age, but those who accepted the invitation but then did not attend reported more health problems overall, both physical and psychological. The differences were especially marked for emotional distress, social isolation and sleep problems. Non-attenders thus appear to be a heterogeneous group, and a mixed strategy will be needed if more of them are to be persuaded to attend.

The third project, based in Manchester, has had two main aims: to examine differences between attenders and non-attenders, in much the same way as in the UK TEDBC; and to investigate women's responses to screening once the appointment is over. To tackle the first issue, the authors selected a random sample of all women aged 50–79 who had been invited for screening from two general practices (Hobbs *et al.*, 1980; Hobbs, 1989). An additional sample who had referred themselves were included as well, and both groups were interviewed after they had attended for their appointment or had failed to appear.

The following results emerged: women who accepted their invitation were on average younger than those who rejected it, but self-referers were younger still; self-referers were from higher social classes on average than those who were invited, but there was no difference between acceptors and rejectors in the invited groups; acceptors were more likely than rejectors to believe that cancer could be cured; acceptors were somewhat more likely than rejectors to have used health screening before, notably cervical smears, chest X-rays and dental checks, and self-referers were more likely still; and, while self-selectors were the most likely to report a personal or family history of breast disease, there was no difference between acceptors and rejectors.

The second part of the Manchester project has been concerned with women's responses to screening once they have attended, particularly their satisfaction with the service they receive (Eardley and Elkind, 1990; Elkind and Eardley, 1990). The NHS Breast Screening Programme has developed a set of guidelines for improving the acceptability of screening (Gray and Austoker, 1988), and there are three central goals: to achieve high coverage nationally; to promote satisfaction; and to minimize anxiety. The purpose of the Manchester study was to find out the 'baseline' against which improvements would have to be measured.

The Manchester unit was one of the first to be set up under the national initiative that followed the Forrest Report – so-called Forrest Units – and the study examined some of the earliest attenders. From one target group practice, 304 women were invited to attend and, of the 198 who did, 146 completed questionnaires. In addition, all members of the District Health Authority staff aged 50–64 were also invited, a total of 224, and 84 of those completed questionnaires, giving 146 group practice subjects and 84 health professionals. The questionnaire covered just two sides of paper, and asked for open-ended comments on seven areas: the invitation leaflet and covering letter; motives for attending; practical problems getting to the clinic; the facilities at the clinic; having the X-ray taken; negative features of the clinic; and likelihood of attending again if invited in three years' time. The comments were coded and counts were made of the most frequent responses.

The overall level of satisfaction was high for both groups: the invitation was received gratefully, few women had practical problems reaching the clinic or keeping their appointment, and the large majority commented favourably on the clinic and its facilities. There was, however, one important negative finding, and it concerned discomfort and pain. Although no direct question had been included, 21 per cent of the group practice women and 34 per cent of the health professionals reported that having the X-ray taken caused them discomfort – though sometimes only slight – and 5 per cent and 13 per cent reported frank pain.

For the X-ray to be satisfactory technically, the breasts have to be compressed, and the plates themselves sometimes have sharp corners. Stomper *et al.* (1988) had already reported that 11 per cent of women experienced 'moderate or greater discomfort', while Jackson, Lex and Smith (1988) had noted that 11 per cent found the procedures 'very uncomfortable' and 3 per cent 'intolerable', but the present figures were higher still, especially for health professionals. The worry, of course, is that women will be deterred from attending again and will perhaps deter others too. In fact, all but a few in the present study said they *would* attend again in three years' time if they were invited, but the response may not always be so encouraging (Orton *et al.*, 1991).

Improvements to X-ray machinery are being made continually and, in addition, it may be possible to warn women about compression. However, the issue of discomfort and pain will have to be taken seriously. In our own investigation, which we shall describe in the next section, we examine the issue in detail. The existing literature has questioned women *retrospectively*, after they have attended and, since expectations may play an important part in eventual satisfaction, it has been impossible to disentangle the real effects of the procedures themselves from psychological factors. To overcome the problem, our own research uses a prospective design, in which expectations are measured before attendance, and outcome is measured afterwards.

A programme of research

From the previous sections, it has become clear that the best hope for effective population screening is X-ray mammography. Success can be achieved, however, only if rates of attendance are high. The experimental programme now in operation in Britain has set 70 per cent as its minimum acceptable level of attendance, and three main questions arise: Will 70 per cent be reached? What influences a woman to attend or not attend? And, if she does attend, how will she respond to the experience? Our own research addresses all three of the issues, and began in 1988, just as the national programme was starting. The project was funded by the South-East Thames Regional Health Authority and the National Breast Screening Programme of the National Health Service, and the two studies were completed recently. The first examined attendance and satisfaction, and the second concentrated on complaints of discomfort and pain.

Main study: attendance and satisfaction

Design and sample

The first of our studies – the main study – was conducted in the South-East Thames Regional Health Authority, and used a prospective design (Figure 3.5) (Vaile *et al.*, 1993). The first phase examined attendance. Some two weeks before they received their invitation for screening, women were sent our Time 1 questionnaire. The invitation came from the local breast screening co-ordinators, and the questionnaire came from us. The invitation was timed to arrive 2–4 weeks before the screening appointment to allow the woman to change the date and time if she wished. To those who had not replied, reminder questionnaires were sent out two weeks and four weeks after the first was posted.

The follow-up phase of the study examined satisfaction with the service. Women who completed the first postal questionnaire, attended for screening and received a negative result were sent a second postal questionnaire as soon as was convenient after they had received their result. The group included women who had been referred back for a second screen because of technical problems with the X-ray and whose result was confirmed as negative, but it excluded women whose result was positive. The

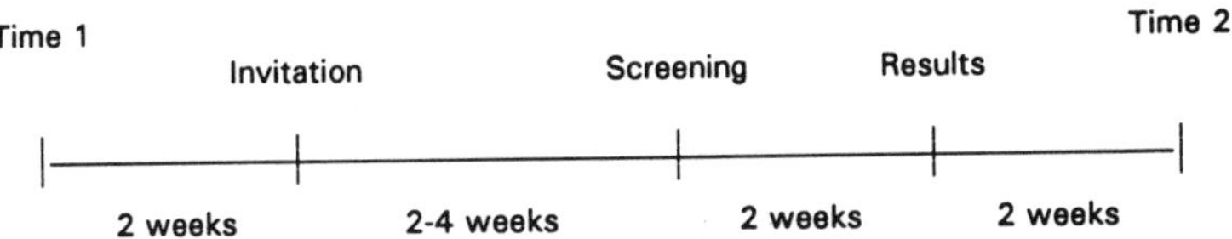

Figure 3.5 Main study: design

questionnaire invited the woman to comment on all aspects of the service, and asked what had made her decide to be screened, what practical difficulties if any she had had in getting to the clinic, what she had thought of the staff and facilities there, and how she had felt about the X-ray itself, including whether it had caused discomfort or pain. We also asked about satisfaction with the service and whether the woman thought she would return in three years' time when she was invited again.

There are known to be marked differences across the country in rates of attendance, no doubt attributable in part to differences in the way the services are organized and in the demographic constitution of the local population. We therefore chose to base our research in three locations, each with rather different characteristics: one rural (Canterbury and Thanet), one provincial (Brighton and Eastbourne) and one inner city (Lewisham in London).

From the lists prepared by the Family Health Services Authority, screening co-ordinators make up 'batches' of women according to locality and invite them for screening when the mammography unit is to be near their home. The unit is normally a mobile 'caravan', which parks at a particular site for 3–6 months. For each of our locations we selected whole batches, which typically contain 1,000–1,200 women. The criterion for which batches to select was simply the convenience of our own timetable.

Questionnaires were sent to 3,160 women at Time 1 (excluding mistaken mailings attributable to inaccuracies in the registers and changes of address) (Figure 3.6). Of the 3,160, 2,060 (65 per cent) responded to the questionnaire: 853 out of 1,182 (72 per cent) in the rural area, 702 out of 1,057 (66 per cent) in the provincial area, and 505 out of 921 (55 per cent) in the inner city area. Attendance averaged 72 per cent (2,275 out of the 3,160): 896 out of 1,182 (76 per cent) in the rural area, 800 out of 1,057 (76 per cent) in the provincial area, and 579 out of 921 (63 per cent) in the inner city area – figures which were similar to those at corresponding times when the study was not in progress. Attendance among responders to the Time 1 questionnaire was uniformly high and averaged 84 per cent (1,728 out of 2,060). Of the 1,728 possible subjects at Time 2, 1,528 completed the follow-up questionnaire (88 per cent): 91 per cent for the rural area, 88

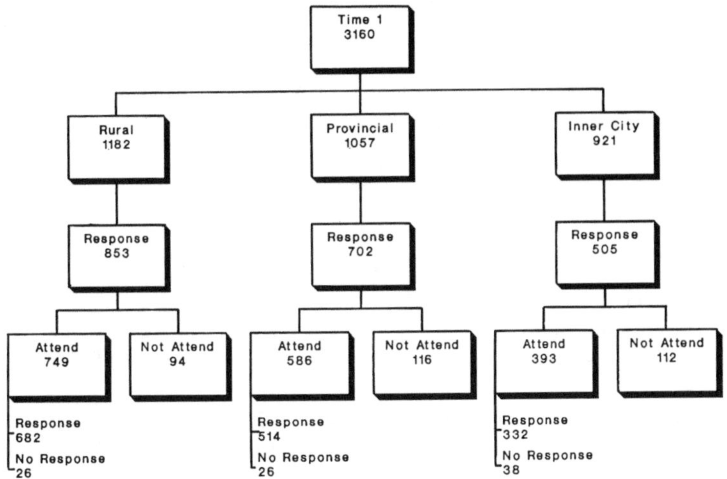

Figure 3.6 Main study: subjects and design

per cent for the provincial area, and 85 per cent for the inner city area.

The characteristics of the women who responded at Time 1 are shown in Table 3.2, and there were noticeable differences between the three areas, as we expected. More women in the provincial area were middle-class than in the other two areas; more in the rural area were married than in the other areas; and more in the inner city area reported poor health and recent illness than those in the other areas, while fewer had had a cervical smear, a mammogram or a clinical breast examination.

Questionnaires

The purpose of the Time 1 questionnaire was twofold: to identify variables that would predict attendance and non-attendance; and to explore the possibility that characteristics of respondents at Time 1 would help to explain their responses at Time 2. All instruments and procedures were tested in a pilot study of 300 women in Canterbury, and the main study used the refined versions.

The questionnaire was divided into four sections (Table 3.3).

Table 3.2 Main study: Demography, health status, and health behaviour, by district

	Rural (853)		Provincial (702)		Inner City (505)		Chi^2
	N	%	N	%	N	%	
Age							
up to 55	367	43.0	317	45.2	250	49.6	5.5
56 plus	486	57.0	385	54.8	254	50.4	
Education							
some qualifications	390	45.7	326	46.4	217	43.1	1.5
no qualifications	463	54.3	376	53.6	287	56.9	
Class							
middle-class	390	59.5	401	69.1	254	59.8	14.6 ***
working-class	265	40.5	179	30.9	171	40.2	
Marriage							
married	666	79.1	501	72.3	345	69.1	18.6 ***
other	176	20.9	192	27.7	154	30.9	
Recent health							
good	625	73.3	489	69.7	309	61.3	21.4 ***
not good	228	26.7	213	30.3	195	38.7	
Recent illness							
yes	272	32.5	257	37.0	219	44.7	19.7 ***
no/unsure	565	67.5	438	63.0	271	55.3	
Previous smear							
yes	755	88.5	636	90.6	427	84.7	9.9 **
no/unsure	98	11.5	66	9.4	77	15.3	
Previous mammogram							
yes	262	30.7	163	23.2	113	22.4	16.0 ***
no/unsure	591	69.3	539	76.8	391	77.6	
Previous breast exam							
yes	386	45.3	408	58.1	207	41.4	40.7 ***
no/unsure	467	54.7	294	41.9	297	58.9	

** $p < 0.01$
*** $p < 0.001$

The first, ‘Keeping Healthy’, asked about the woman’s current health and her previous use of cervical cytology and breast examinations, including X-ray mammography. The second, ‘Breast Screening’, was based on the Theory of Planned

Table 3.3 Main study: The Time 1 questionnaire

Keeping Healthy
- Current health
- Previous cervical cytology
- Previous breast screening and examinations

Breast Screening
- Attitude to being screened
- Perceived behavioural control
- Expectations about breast screening

Breast Cancer
- Perceived vulnerability to breast cancer
- History of breast abnormalities
- Factual knowledge about breast cancer

Some Details about You
- Age
- Marriage
- Education
- Social class

Behaviour (Ajzen, 1988), an extension of the Theory of Reasoned Action we discussed in Chapter 1, and measured the woman's attitude to having her breasts screened and her subjective norm about being screened (Figure 3.7). There were ten items for beliefs, ten for outcome evaluations, five for normative beliefs, and five for motivation to comply. All were measured on five-point scales from 'Strongly Disagree' to 'Strongly Agree', and beliefs, normative beliefs and motivation to comply were scaled from 1 to 5, while outcome evaluations were scaled from -2 to $+2$, the positive pole denoting positive views.[2] Attitude is the sum of the belief *x* outcome evaluation products, and subjective norm is the sum of the normative belief *x*

2. Fishbein and Ajzen (1975) at different points in their book recommend unipolar and bipolar scaling for outcome evaluation. In line with several recent authors (reviewed by Hewstone and Young, 1988) we favour bipolar scales.

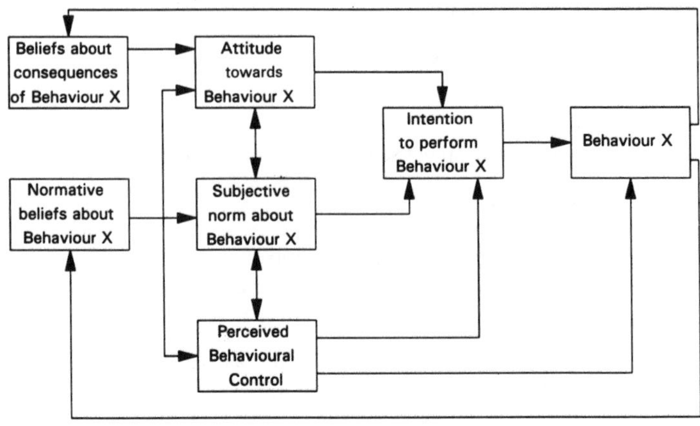

Figure 3.7 Theory of planned behaviour. Source: Ajzen (1988), reprinted by permission of Open University Press.

motivation to comply products. Cronbach's alpha for attitude was 0.76 and for subjective norm it was 0.86.

Two other sets of questions were included in the 'Breast Screening' section. The first measured what Ajzen (1988) has called 'perceived behavioural control'. Women may intend to accept their invitation for screening, but may acknowledge even at the time of receipt that uncontrollable events may overtake them and prevent attendance – illness, holidays, lack of transport, for example. Some women may thus believe they have little control over what their eventual behaviour will be, while others believe they have great control. Ajzen argues that perceived behavioural control may work alongside attitude and subjective norm to influence intention and so behaviour, or it may affect behaviour directly, but either way it will be an important predictor of behaviour. Three items were therefore included, and Cronbach's alpha was 0.77. The remaining questions in the section were about expectations of what would happen at the appointment, and they all offered a choice of responses from which the woman was asked to select one.

Section 3, 'Breast Cancer', asked a variety of additional questions about breast cancer, both factual and attitudinal, including whether the woman had experienced problems with her breasts in the past and how vulnerable to the disease she felt herself to be. Perceived vulnerability was measured by the five vulnerability items from Stillman's perceived vulnerability and severity scale (Stillman, 1977), and Cronbach's alpha was found to be 0.60, but only after the fifth item was removed. The final section of the questionnaire, 'Some Details About You', asked for demographic information – age, education, marital status and social class. At the very end there was a box for respondents' comments.

The postal questionnaire at Time 2 for attenders was much shorter, and was designed to tap the woman's reactions to screening, from the time she received her invitation to the time she received her result. Some of the questions asked for open-ended responses, and others were divided into subsidiary questions, each with a five-point scale. Since one of our main interests was respondents' satisfaction, the seven separate items for satisfaction were combined to make a scale. Cronbach's alpha was 0.89.

Characteristics of attenders

The first question to address in our data was whether attenders differed from non-attenders. Four sets of characteristics were examined: social inputs (which meant demographic characteristics in the present study), health status and health behaviours, expectations about screening and attitudes towards screening. Our first analysis examined social inputs and found that they played little part (Table 3.4). The only significant finding for the whole sample combined was that married women were more likely to attend than those who were single, widowed, separated or divorced. Most of the effect was due to the women in the provincial area. In contrast to demographic characteristics, health status and health behaviour had important effects. Women with good health were more likely to attend than those with poor health, as were those with no long-standing illness and those who had had a cervical smear or clinical breast examination at some time in the past. Women who had had a mammogram, however, were less likely to attend than those who had not, in general because they had only recently had one and so were not yet due for another. In each case, the finding for the whole sample

Table 3.4 Main study: Attendance by demography, health status and health behaviour

	Rural % attended	Provincial % attended	Inner City % attended	Whole Sample % attended
Age				
up to 55	88.3	83.6	76.4	83.5
56 plus	88.1	82.3	79.5	84.2
Education				
some qualifications	85.4 *	82.8	76.5	82.4
no qualifications	90.5	83.0	79.1	85.1
Class				
middle-class	86.9	83.3	75.6	82.8
working-class	90.2	84.9	78.9	85.5
Marriage				
married	89.5	86.2 ***	77.1	85.6 **
other	84.7	75.5	79.9	79.9
Recent health				
good	88.2	84.5	82.5 **	85.7 ***
not good	88.2	79.3	70.8	79.9
Recent illness				
yes	87.5	80.2	74.9	81.3 *
no/unsure	88.5	84.7	80.4	85.5
Previous smear				
yes	89.8 ***	84.6 ***	78.7	85.4 ***
no/unsure	75.5	66.7	74.0	72.6
Previous mammogram				
yes	82.8 **	67.5 ***	66.4 ***	74.7 ***
no/unsure	90.5	87.6	81.3	87.1
Previous breast exam				
yes	90.2	85.5 *	81.6	86.5 **
no/unsure	86.5	79.3	75.4	81.4

* $p < 0.05$
** $p < 0.01$
*** $p < 0.001$
Attendance rates: Rural 87.8% Provincial 83.5% Inner City 77.8% Whole Sample 83.9%
Significance levels are for 2 × 2 Chi^2 tests.

combined was consistent across all three areas considered separately.

The next analysis examined expectations. Women who expected to have to wait a long time at the centre (over 30 minutes) and who thought screening itself would take a long time (over 20 minutes) were less likely to attend than those who expected greater speed, but how long the result was expected to take to arrive had no effect. Expectations that the staff would not answer questions or explain the procedures were strongly associated with non-attendance, but whether the staff were expected to explain the possible results had no effect. Who would do the screening and whether the procedure would be carried out in a private room also had no effect.

The remaining analysis of attendance examined attitudes towards attending for screening. According to Ajzen's Theory of Planned Behaviour, attendance will be predicted by three things: a positive attitude towards attending for screening, a positive subjective norm towards it and a positive feeling of perceived control over attendance. All three scales, it emerged, had marked effects on attendance (Table 3.5), which was predicted by a positive attitude, a positive subjective norm, a positive perception of one's control over attendance, and also a feeling of vulnerability to breast cancer. The measures were much the strongest predictors of all those we examined and they showed consistency across all three areas.

Response to the service

Once women had attended for screening, our focus shifted from why they had attended to how they responded to the service they received. Items were combined where possible into scales, and Cronbach's alphas were as follows: 0.73 for the invitation letter and leaflet, 0.68 for the facilities at the centre, 0.88 for the staff and 0.89 for overall satisfaction with the experience. All four scales were standardized to run from 1 to 5. Discomfort, pain and intention to return were each measured by a single five-point scale.

There was considerable satisfaction with the service in all three areas, it emerged, and almost all the respondents said they would return when they were invited again in three years' time. Satisfaction averaged 4.5 on our five-point scale for the whole sample combined (4.6 rural, 4.4 provincial, 4.3 inner city), and

Table 3.5 Main study: Attendance by attitudes

	Attend		Not Attend			
	Mean	SD	Mean	SD	d.f.	t
Rural	N = 749		N = 94			
attitude	28.9	15.0	23.3	18.3	841	3.4 ***
subjective norm	67.2	23.8	54.8	24.9	778	4.7 ***
perceived control	13.0	1.9	12.0	2.6	843	4.7 ***
perceived vulnerability	16.3	3.5	15.5	3.3	842	2.1 *
Provincial	N = 586		N = 116			
attitude	30.1	15.5	22.0	17.5	694	5.0 ***
subjective norm	63.2	23.3	53.4	26.2	646	3.9 ***
perceived control	13.1	1.7	12.4	2.3	687	4.0 ***
perceived vulnerability	16.4	3.4	15.4	4.3	688	3.0 **
Inner city	N = 393		N = 112			
attitude	29.2	15.5	24.7	17.6	489	2.6 *
subjective norm	62.9	24.3	53.5	27.1	452	3.3 ***
perceived control	12.8	2.0	11.6	3.1	489	4.8 ***
perceived vulnerability	16.1	3.7	14.5	4.9	494	3.7 ***
Whole sample	N = 1728		N = 322			
attitude	29.4	15.3	23.3	17.8	2028	6.3 ***
subjective norm	64.9	23.8	53.9	26.0	1880	7.1 ***
perceived control	13.0	1.8	12.0	2.7	2023	8.0 ***
perceived vulnerability	16.3	3.5	15.1	4.2	2028	5.4 ***

* $p < 0.05$
** $p < 0.01$
*** $p < 0.001$

94.6 per cent of the combined sample said they would return (96.5 per cent rural, 92.8 per cent provincial, 93.3 per cent inner city). Large numbers of women, however, reported discomfort, or even pain, despite what they had said about satisfaction and intention to return: discomfort 40 per cent of the sample overall, and pain 13 per cent.

Our next concern was to try to *predict* satisfaction. The first of the analyses examined the effects of demographic characteristics, health status and health behaviour. There were just two: women who were married reported greater satisfaction in the combined sample and the rural sample than those who were single, widowed, separated or divorced; and those who had had a recent illness reported less satisfaction than those who had not. Expectations also had two effects, both of them to do with the staff: satisfaction was lowest among women who had expected the staff not to answer questions and not to explain the procedures.

The strongest of our predictors were to emerge from the attitudes we had measured at Time 1 and the way the women perceived their experience once it was over. The effects for all the measures in combination were examined by multiple regression, for each of the areas separately and for the whole sample together. The leading predictors were the facilities at the centre and, for two of the three areas, the behaviour of the staff. Attitudes played different roles in different areas – subjective norm was a significant predictor in the rural area, attitude in the provincial area and attitude and perceived behavioural control in the inner city area. Response to the invitation leaflet and letter had no effects, but the time it took the result to arrive predicted satisfaction (negatively) in the inner city area and in the sample taken as a whole. Discomfort and pain played no significant part in any of the three areas, but both reached statistical significance as negative predictors of satisfaction in the combined sample. The proportions of variance explained by the significant predictor variables in combination were substantial – 23 per cent in the rural area, 24 per cent in the provincial area and 39 per cent in the inner city area – and for the combined sample the figure was 30 per cent.

Analyses of the sort we have presented so far provide a detailed *description* of findings, but they do not allow one to combine the data theoretically, in such a way that an examination can be made of mechanisms and patterns of mediation. For that, we turned to hierarchical regression and path analysis. The first stage of the new analyses was to posit a model of the possible relationships between variables (Figure 3.8). Our model begins with social inputs (demographic characteristics). Social inputs, we propose, influence both current health status and previous health behaviours, which in turn lead to attitudes and expectations

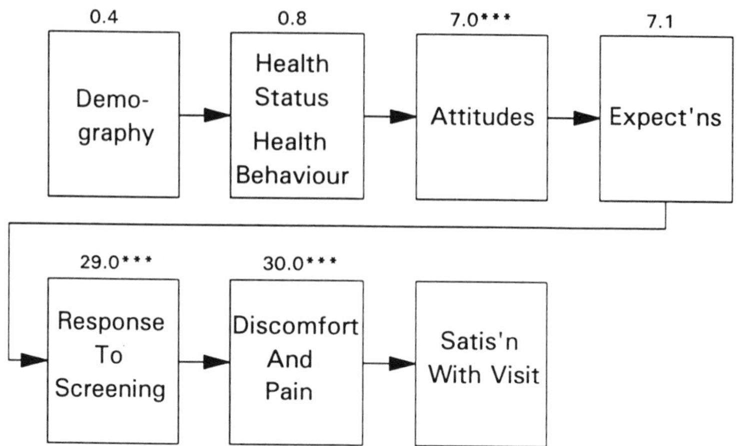

Figure 3.8 Main study: hierarchical analysis for satisfaction. (*** $p < 0.001$)

about screening. Attitudes and expectations at Time 1 will be important influences on how women respond to screening – staff, facilities, discomfort, pain – and those responses in turn will influence overall satisfaction with the visit. The model is hierarchical and considers the causal ordering of *blocks* of variables. By the subsequent use of path analysis, it was possible to 'open' the boxes and examine the role of *individual* variables and so to produce a 'map' of the causal links among them.

The first analysis we conducted was a hierarchical analysis of satisfaction for the whole sample combined (Figure 3.8). Thirty per cent of the variance was explained altogether, and the blocks that made a significant contribution were discomfort and pain, response to the screening session itself and attitudes. Reading from the start of our model, demographic characteristics and health status and behaviour made no contribution, but attitudes explained 7 per cent of the variance. Expectations made no further contribution to the cumulative variance explained, but response to screening added 22 per cent. Discomfort and pain added another 1 per cent which, though a small increment, nevertheless reached statistical significance.

Our second analysis was a path analysis of satisfaction, based on repeated multiple regression analyses, again for the whole sample combined (Figure 3.9). There are four points to make. First, the most important predictors of satisfaction were the way the woman responded to the staff and to the facilities at the unit – in part, no doubt, a reflection of objective characteristics. There were two other predictors, both of them negative: the time it took the woman's result to arrive and discomfort experienced during the X-ray. Second, both response to staff and response to facilities were influenced by the attitude the woman *brought to* her screening appointment, and response to facilities was influenced by subjective norm too. Perceived vulnerability to breast cancer played no part; nor did expectations. Third, attitude was unrelated to health status, but previous experience of mammography led to a negative attitude, while experience of other clinical examinations led to a positive attitude. Experience of clinical breast examinations was related to social class in that clinical examinations were more common among middle-class women than working-class women. Fourth, discomfort played a pivotal role in that it mediated the effects upon satisfaction of education, social class, previous clinical breast examination and time to receive the result. That is, educated, middle-class women

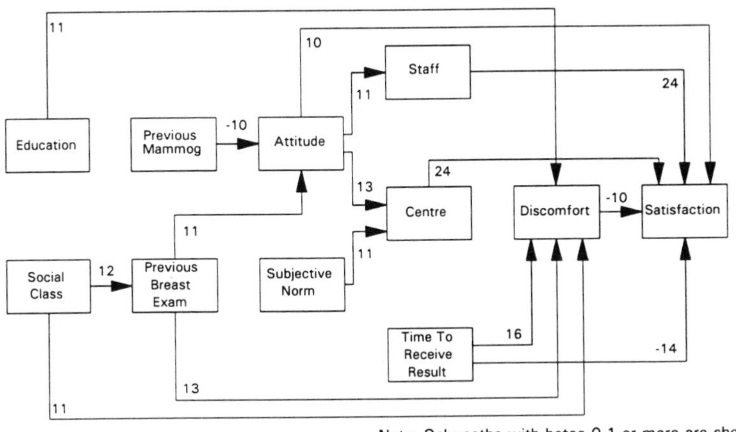

Figure 3.9 Main study: path analysis for satisfaction

reported discomfort more than did women without educational qualifications and from working-class backgrounds, and discomfort was greatest in women who had had clinical breast examinations before and who had had to wait a long time for their present result to arrive. These last results in particular have important implications for policy and practice, and we shall return to discuss them at the end of the chapter.

Conclusion

The first aim of the main study was to predict attendance, and we succeeded. Social inputs were relatively unimportant in that there were no differences by social class, though attenders *were* more likely than non-attenders to be married. The pattern was similar to that from the only other study we know to have used a prospective design (Calnan and Chamberlain, 1984; Calnan, 1984b) and might be explained by the influence of social support in encouraging women to use screening services. Alternatively it may simply be that more of the women who were not married were at work and had difficulty keeping daytime appointments. Current health status, we found, and previous health behaviour both had a number of effects on attendance, while expectations did not. Much the strongest predictors, however, were attitudes, for the woman's attitude, her subjective norm, and her perceived control over attendance all predicted attendance strongly. So too did the belief that she was susceptible to breast cancer, though to a lesser extent.

The second aim of the study was to examine satisfaction with the service and to try to predict it from the variety of measures we explored. Demographic characteristics, health status, health behaviour and expectations all had little effect, it emerged. Attitudes, in contrast, did have significant effects, but it was overwhelmingly the behaviour of the staff and the facilities at the centre that mattered most. The important aspects of behaviour were how well the staff explained things and answered questions, and how friendly, reassuring and efficient they were; and the important aspects of the centre were how well it was designed and run, and how welcoming (or non-frightening) it was. As in the previous literature, the overall level of satisfaction was consistently high throughout our study, but there were two important 'negative' findings: many women had to wait two weeks or more for their result to arrive; and substantial numbers complained that screening was uncomfortable and even painful. Discomfort proved to be a pivotal mediator of satisfaction in our path analysis, and it has become a matter of concern to the national Forrest programme. There were a number of important issues about discomfort and pain to explore further, we believed, and we therefore designed a follow-up study, to which we now turn.

Follow-up study: discomfort and pain

The main study revealed that over 40 per cent of women complained of discomfort during mammography, and 13 per cent complained of frank pain. There were marked differences between the three areas – for example, discomfort was reported by under 30 per cent of respondents in the rural area but almost 60 per cent in the inner city – and a wide range of values have been reported in the published literature, as we saw earlier in the chapter. The immediate practical concern is that discomfort may discourage future attendance, and we believed it was therefore important to examine the issues in some detail, in a way that had not been possible in the main study. There were four main objectives: to confirm the proportion of women who report discomfort and pain; to measure the quality of the discomfort or pain; to try to predict attendance and reported discomfort; and to examine the implications of our findings for modifying screening procedures and perhaps for improving health education and promotion.

Design and procedure

The design of the study was again prospective and the sample came from a single 'batch' in Maidstone, a rural health district in the South East Thames Regional Health Authority (Rutter *et al.*, 1992). All the women were to be screened in a mobile unit. At Time 1, shortly before the invitation to screening was to be sent out, 1,160 women received a postal questionnaire from us. The questions were designed to tap a variety of areas, many of them the same as in the main study: the respondent's current health status and previous health behaviours, including attendance for cervical screening and mammography; her trait and state anxiety levels, measured by Spielberger's State-Trait Anxiety Inventory (Spielberger, Gorsuch and Lushene, 1970); whether she intended to accept the invitation to attend and what obstacles to attendance she foresaw; her expectations about the procedures and the staff; her knowledge and beliefs about breast cancer, including how vulnerable she perceived herself to be; background demographic information; and information about her physical build, including weight and bust measurement.

Of the 1,160 women we approached, 774 completed the questionnaire (67 per cent), and 617 of the 774 attended (80 per cent) (Figure 3.10). At Time 2, which was immediately after the woman had dressed at the end of her screen, an 'interviewer' sat with her and asked her to complete a three-sided questionnaire

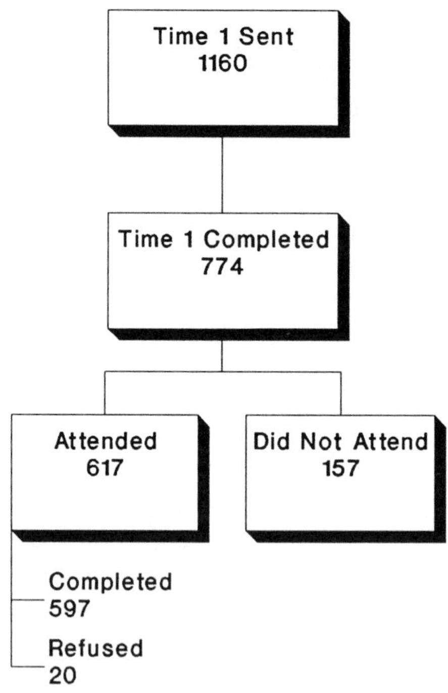

Figure 3.10 Pain study: subjects and design

about her experiences. The questions covered (1) whether she had experienced discomfort or pain during the procedures; (2) whether she was still experiencing discomfort or pain at the time of completing the questionnaire; (3) how her experience compared with the discomfort she had expected from screening and had felt during other medical procedures; and (4) how she would characterize whatever pain she had felt, using a series of sixteen adjectives we provided from the McGill Pain Inventory (Melzack, 1975). There were two additional measures: whether the woman was pleased she had attended for screening; and whether she intended to return when she received her next invitation in three years' time. Of the 774 women who attended, all but 20 completed the Time 2 questionnaire (97 per cent response rate).

Extent of discomfort

Figure 3.11 shows the levels of discomfort and pain. Discomfort was experienced by 34.5 per cent of the women during the mammography itself, and 6.2 per cent reported pain. By the time

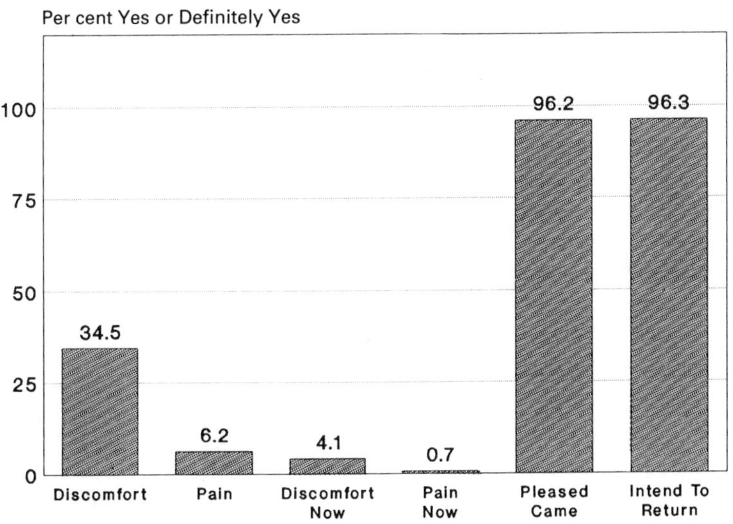

Figure 3.11 Pain study: discomfort and pain

the questionnaire was completed between 5 and 10 minutes after the screen, the figures had fallen to 4.1 per cent and 0.7 per cent respectively. All but 4 per cent of the women said they were pleased they had attended and intended to return next time. The important points were thus that the levels of discomfort and pain during the procedures were close to the rural average in the main study, that within 5 or 10 minutes of the X-ray they had fallen very considerably, and that virtually all the respondents were pleased they had attended and said they would return. Correlations between discomfort and pain on the one hand and satisfaction on the other were small and accounted for no more than 5 per cent of the variance.

Characteristics of discomfort

Figure 3.12 shows the comparisons the respondents drew between the discomfort they experienced and what they had expected during screening and had experienced during other medical procedures. For 67.8 per cent of the sample, the discomfort of screening was 'less' or 'much less' than they had

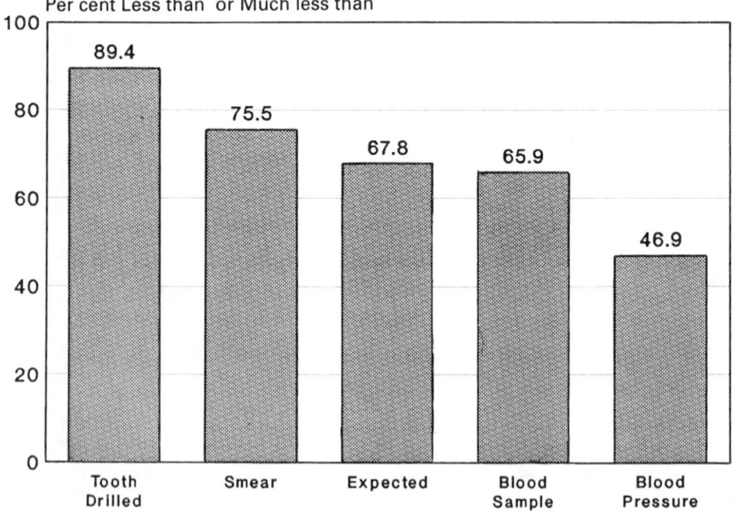

Figure 3.12 Pain study: comparisons of discomfort

expected. For 89.4 per cent it was 'less' or 'much less' than the discomfort of having a tooth drilled, and the figures for the other comparisons were 75.5 per cent for having a cervical smear, 65.9 per cent for giving a blood sample, and 46.9 per cent for having one's blood pressure taken. Put another way, in rank order, having a tooth drilled was the most likely to produce discomfort, followed by having a cervical smear, giving a blood sample, undergoing mammography, and finally having one's blood pressure taken. Mammography was thus 'preferable' to all but the last. The adjectives respondents used most frequently to describe the pain they had felt were 'crushing' and 'tender', but the proportion of women who reported moderate or severe pain on the other dimensions was generally no more than 2 per cent (Figure 3.13).

Predictors of attendance and discomfort

The last of our analyses tested whether attendance and reported discomfort at Time 2 could be predicted from any of the measures we had taken at Time 1: physical build, demographic

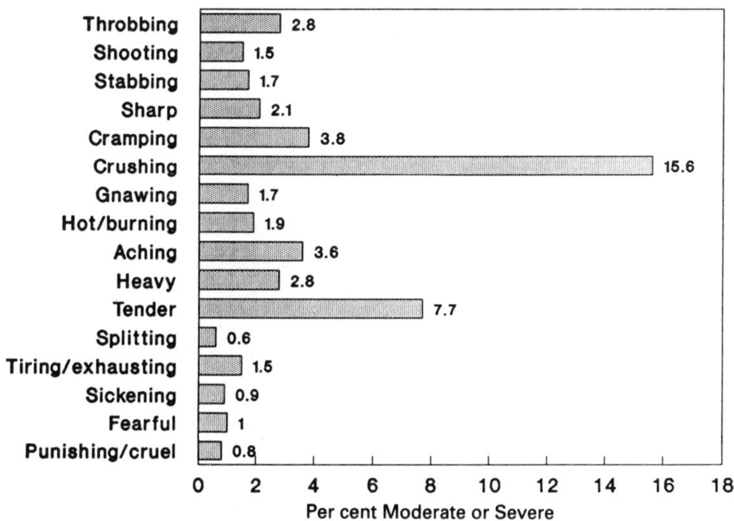

Figure 3.13 Pain study: descriptions of pain

inputs, current health status and previous health behaviours, anxiety and perceived vulnerability to breast cancer, expectations about the procedures and intention to attend. Attendance was predicted by four measures: having had a cervical smear in the past; having had no recent mammogram; expecting the procedure would not cause discomfort; and expecting the procedure would not cause pain. For discomfort, again there were four predictors: having educational qualifications; having experience of previous clinical breast examinations; and expecting that the X-ray would cause discomfort or would cause pain (Table 3.6). The effect of education was to be expected since it is common in the literature on medical interventions, and the effect of previous experience of clinical breast examinations probably occurred because examinations other than mammography cause little discomfort and can lead to unduly optimistic expectations about mammography. What we had not foreseen were the effects for expectations about discomfort and pain, especially pain, for two-thirds of women who reported discomfort had said at Time 1 that they expected the procedure to cause pain, against only one-third who had said they did not expect pain. Of all the measures we took, the *expectation* of pain thus proved to be the most important: it separated attenders from non-attenders; and it distinguished women who reported discomfort from those who did not.

Conclusion

The first aim of the follow-up study was to establish the extent of discomfort and pain. Discomfort during the X-ray was reported by 34.5 per cent of respondents, and 6.2 per cent reported frank pain – figures that were very similar to those for the rural area in the main study. Within 5 or 10 minutes of the X-ray, however, the figures had fallen to 4.1 per cent and 0.7 per cent, an indication that the effects were generally short-lived and perhaps less worrying for the service than previous investigators may have implied.

The second aim of the study was to ask respondents to characterize the discomfort they had experienced, and two techniques were used: comparisons with the effects of other medical interventions and descriptions using a standard set of adjectives. The comparisons revealed that mammography caused

Table 3.6 Pain study: Time 1 predictors of reported discomfort

	% discomfort/unsure
Education	
qualifications	42.9 **
no qualifications	31.1
Previous breast examination	
yes	41.0 *
no/unsure	31.9
Discomfort expected	
yes	43.9 *
no/unsure	34.2
Pain expected	
yes	65.6 ***
no/unsure	35.0

* $p < 0.05$
** $p < 0.01$
*** $p < 0.001$
There were no effects for physical build, health status, anxiety or perceived vulnerability to cancer. Discomfort correlated − 0.14 *** with overall satisfaction and − 0.15 *** with intention to return in three years' time. Satisfaction and intention to return correlated + 0.83 ***.

less discomfort than expected for two-thirds of respondents, and ranked much like having one's blood pressure taken. For the majority of women, giving a blood sample, having a cervical smear and having a tooth drilled all caused more discomfort than mammography.

The third aim of the study was to try to predict attendance and reported discomfort from the measures we had taken at Time 1 – measures of physical build, demographic social inputs, current health status and previous health behaviours, and anxiety and expectations. Just two measures predicted both attendance and reported discomfort: expectations about discomfort and expectations about pain. As we concluded in our previous study, what the woman *brings to* mammography, psychologically, is of greater importance than anything else we have measured, and in this case the significant part of what she brought was her expectations.

Implications for theory, policy and practice

In this final section of the chapter, we draw out the implications of our investigation for theory and for policy and practice. The implications for theory concern the role of social inputs and psychological measures for predicting outcome, the value of the concept of mediation, and the significance of prospective research designs. The implications for policy and practice concern the organization of services, the importance of staff and facilities at mammography centres, the debate about discomfort and pain, and the contribution to be made to mammography by health education and promotion.

Implications for theory

The first theoretical implication of our findings is that social psychological variables do play a part, as we predicted, in breast screening. First, women who attended for screening in the main study had more positive attitudes, subjective norms and perceived control over attendance than women who did not attend, and they also felt somewhat more vulnerable to breast cancer. Second, women who came away from their X-ray saying they were satisfied with the service had generally reported a more positive attitude at Time 1 and greater perceived control over attendance. Third, expectations that screening would be painful emerged in the follow-up study as significant predictors of both attendance and outcome: it discouraged attendance and encouraged reported discomfort. Throughout the investigation, social psychological measures have produced some of the strongest and most reliable results, in a way that previous research has not made clear.

The second implication of our findings concerns the concept of mediation. In Chapter 1, we outlined a model of health which argues that relationships between inputs and outcomes are most usefully viewed as *mediated* through social psychological and other variables. That is, social inputs such as education and class, and health inputs such as previous use of screening services – which are known to be associated with a wide range of health outcomes – influence those outcomes *through* variables such as attitudes and expectations. The present investigation has produced good evidence for our approach, particularly in the analyses of satisfaction in the main study. To take just one example, middle-class women reported more discomfort than working-class women. By examining the paths of mediation, we were able to show that part of the effect occurred because middle-class women were more likely than working-class women to have had a previous clinical breast examination. Clinical examinations encourage women to have a positive attitude towards mammography but also to report discomfort, in part because clinical methods generally cause little discomfort and so may raise expectations for mammography which in the event are disappointed. To conclude that middle-class women report discomfort more than working-class women is less useful theoretically – and indeed practically – than to go on to say why. A model of mediation allows one to take that extra step.

The third implication of our findings is that we have confirmed the value of prospective designs in research of this sort. Prospective designs allow one to use measures taken at one point in a longitudinal study to predict later outcomes: there is no contamination and no resort to retrospective measures of earlier variables. Only in prospective designs can longitudinal effects and mediation be measured with confidence.

Implications for policy and practice

The first implication of our findings for policy and practice concerns the organization of screening services in this country. There are three points. First, we found evidence that the registers of women kept by the Family Health Service Authorities were inaccurate. The most common problem was that addresses were out of date – normally because the woman had moved away, but on occasion because the house no longer even existed. The inaccuracies were greatest in the inner city area, where almost 10 per cent of questionnaires at Time 1 were returned to us by the Post Office or new occupants because the woman was not known at the address. The FHSA register is the foundation of the entire Forrest programme: the greater its inaccuracy, the less the effectiveness of the programme.

The second point is the time it takes for the woman to receive her result. The range was considerable – over 90 per cent of women in the main study's rural sample heard within a week, against 50 per cent in the inner city area and only 20 per cent in the provincial area – and delay was an important source of dissatisfaction. For women who are recalled, because their screen is inadequate technically or because there is evidence of abnormality which needs further investigation, there is still further delay. Greater speed is necessary if satisfaction and adherence are to be maximized.

The third point is the marked difference between geographical areas in the demographic characteristics of the population. The differences are well known – ethnicity and social class, for example, in inner city versus rural areas – and our investigation revealed marked differences by area in response rate and satisfaction particularly. How to accommodate the differences, in the way one tries to recruit women to be screened and to offer and fund an appropriate service, is a major challenge.

The second implication of our findings for policy and practice concerns staffing and the facilities offered in screening units. From the main study it emerged clearly that friendly, responsive, efficient staff and well-designed, well-run, non-threatening facilities were the leading predictors of satisfaction with the service. Screening takes only 4 or 5 minutes, yet the findings suggest that 4 or 5 minutes is quite long enough to establish a positive relationship with the woman, given high quality staff. Professional education and training must continue to focus on developing skills to enhance the relationship between the professional and the client, and there must be a continued emphasis on providing high quality facilities at centres.

The third implication concerns discomfort and pain. Previous research suggests that many women report discomfort during mammography, and practitioners and administrators in the Forrest programme have begun to see the issues as important. From our own research there are three main points to make. First, although substantial numbers of women did report discomfort, discomfort and pain had all but disappeared within 5 or 10 minutes of screening for all but a very few women. What is more, the discomfort of screening was seen by the majority as noticeably less than the discomfort of other routine medical procedures, for which a degree of discomfort is regarded as acceptable and unavoidable. The implication is that current procedures are satisfactory. Second, reported discomfort had little effect on dissatisfaction. There was, it is true, a *statistical* relationship, but it accounted for less than 5 per cent of the variance and was too small to be of *practical* significance. It will be important to continue to monitor re-attendance rates, but the present evidence suggests that discomfort will play a very small part. Finally, for two-thirds of the women, discomfort was less than they had expected. It is this last point that has the most important implications, for, while most women have no personal experience of mammography and so must build their expectations on whatever information they have available, we have shown that expectations have important effects upon both attendance and reported discomfort. The risk is that the most available and readily recalled information will be used – typically negative reports from newspaper and television features – and that positive reports will be overlooked. Health education and promotion must try to ensure that accurate and representative information is made available and publicized. Relatives and friends who have experienced mammography themselves may have an especially important part to play.

The final implication of our findings extends what we have just said about health education and promotion. One of the important theoretical conclusions from our research is that women's attitudes predict both attendance and satisfaction. Our work was based on Ajzen's Theory of Planned Behaviour, which distinguishes attitude, subjective norm and perceived behavioural control, and all three were found to play significant roles. Sadly, past attempts at persuasion in health have seldom been based on recognizable theoretical foundations – even large and expensive national campaigns – and we suggest that Ajzen's model would provide a valuable starting point, both for breast screening in particular and for health behaviours in general.

References

Ajzen I (1988), *Attitudes, Personality and Behavior*, Milton Keynes: Open University Press.

Andersson I (1989), Mammographic screening of an urban population in Sweden: implications of results from a randomized trial. In G Ziant (Ed.) *Practical Modalities of an Efficient Screening for Breast Cancer in the European Community*, 94–101, Elsevier.

Andersson I, Aspegren K, Janzon L, Landberg T, Lindholm K, Linell F, Ljungberg O, Ranstam J and Sigfusson B (1988), Mammographic screening and mortality from breast cancer: the Malmo mammographic screening trial, *British Medical Journal*, 297, 943–8.

Calnan M (1984a), Explaining participation in programmes for the early detection of breast cancer, *Community Medicine*, 6, 204–9.

Calnan M (1984b), The health belief model and participation in programmes for the early detection of breast cancer: a comparative analysis, *Social Science and Medicine*, 19, 823–30.

Calnan M (1985), An evaluation of the effectiveness of a class teaching breast self-examination, *British Journal of Medical Psychology*, 58, 317–29.

Calnan M W and Chamberlain J (1984), Explaining participation in programmes for the early detection of breast cancer: a comparative analysis, *Epidemiologie et Santé Publique*, 32, 376–82.

Calnan M W, Chamberlain J and Moss S (1983), Compliance with a class teaching breast self examination, *Journal of Epidemiology and Community Health*, 37, 264–70.

Calnan M W and Moss S (1984), The Health Belief Model and compliance with education given at a class in breast self examination, *Journal of Health and Social Behaviour*, 25, 198–210.

Calnan M and Rutter D R (1986a), Preventive health practices and their relationship with socio-demographic characteristics, *Health Education Research*, 1, 247–53.

Calnan M and Rutter D R (1986b), Do health beliefs predict health behaviour? An analysis of breast self-examination, *Social Science and Medicine*, 22, 673–8.

Calnan M and Rutter D R (1988), Do health beliefs predict health behaviour? A follow-up analysis of breast self-examination, *Social Science and Medicine*, 126, 463–5.

Collette H J A, Day N E, Rombach J and de Waard F (1984), Evaluation of screening for breast cancer in a non-randomized study (the DOM project) by means of a case-control study, *Lancet*, 2 June, 1224–6.

Doll R and Peto R (1986), *The Causes of Cancer*, Oxford: Oxford University Press.

Eardley A and Elkind A (1990), A pilot study of attendance for breast cancer screening, *Social Science and Medicine*, 30, 693–9.

Elkind A and Eardley A (1990), Consumer satisfaction with breast screening: a pilot study, *Journal of Public Health Medicine*, 12, 1, 15–18.

Fagerberg G (1989), Optimum interval between mammographic screening examinations for different age groups. In G Ziant (Ed.) *Practical Modalities of an Efficient Screening for Breast Cancer in the European Community*, 27–34, Elsevier.

Fishbein M and Ajzen I (1975), *Belief, Attitude, Intention and Behavior*, Reading, Mass: Addison-Wesley.

Forrest P (1986), *Breast Cancer Screening*, DHSS Report, London: HMSO.

French K, Porter A M D, Robinson S E, McCallum F M, Howie J G R and Roberts M M (1982), Attendance at a breast screening clinic: a problem of administration or attitudes, *British Medical Journal*, 285, 617–20.

Gray J A M and Austoker J (1988), *Draft Guidelines on Improving Acceptability*, NHS, BSP.

Habbema J D F, van Oortmarssen G J, van Putten D J, Lubbe J T and van der Maas P J (1986), Age-specific reduction in breast cancer mortality by screening: an analysis of the results of the Health Insurance Plan of Greater New York study, *Journal of the National Cancer Institute*, 77, 2, 317–20.

Hewstone M and Young L (1988), Expectancy-value models of attitude: measurement and combination of evaluations and beliefs, *Journal of Applied Social Psychology*, 18, 958–71.

Hill D, White V, Jolley D and Mapperson K (1988), Self examination of the breast: is it beneficial? Meta-analysis of studies investigating breast self examination and extent of disease in patients with breast cancer, *British Medical Journal*, 297, 271–5.

Hobbs P (1989), Factors affecting population participation in breast cancer screening. In G Ziant (Ed.) *Practical Modalities of an Efficient Screening for Breast Cancer in the European Community*, 187–95, Elsevier.

Hobbs P, Smith A, George W D and Sellwood R A (1980), Acceptors and rejectors of an invitation to undergo breast screening compared with those who referred themselves, *Journal of Epidemiology and Community Health*, 32, 19–22.

Hunt S, Alexander F and Roberts M M (1988), Attenders and non-attenders at a breast screening clinic: a comparative study, *Public Health*, 102, 3–10.

Hunt S M, McEwen J and McKenna S P (1986), *Measuring Health Status*, London: Croom Helm.

Jackson V P, Lex A M and Smith D J (1988), Patient discomfort during screen-film mammography, *Radiology*, 168, 421–3.

Leathar D S and Roberts M M (1985), Older women's attitudes towards breast disease, self-examination, and screening facilities: implications for communication, *British Medical Journal*, 290, 668–70.

Maclean U, Sinfield D, Klein S and Harden B (1984), Women who decline breast screening, *Journal of Epidemiology and Community Health*, 38, 278–83.

Mant D, Vessey M P, Neil A, McPherson K and Jones L (1987), Breast self-examination and breast cancer stage at diagnosis, *British Journal of Cancer*, 55, 207–211.

Melzack, R (1975), The McGill pain questionnaire: major properties and scoring methods, *Pain*, 1, 277–99.

Miller A B (1988), Screening for breast cancer: a review, *European Journal of Cancer Clinic Oncology*, 24, 1, 49–53.

Orton M, Fitzpatrick R, Fuller A, Mant D, Mlynek C and Thorogood M (1991), Factors affecting women's response to an invitation to attend for a second breast cancer screening examination, *British Journal of General Practice*, 41, 320–3.

Palli D, del Turco M R, Buiatti E, Ciatto S, Crocetti E and Paci E (1989), Time interval since last test in a breast cancer screening programme: a case-control study in Italy, *Journal of Epidemiology and Community Health*, 43, 241–8.

Reidy J and Hoskins O (1988), Controversy over mammography screening, *British Medical Journal*, 297, 932–3.

Roberts M M (1989), Breast screening: time for a rethink?, *British Medical Journal*, 299, 1153–5.

Roberts M M, Alexander F E, Anderson T J, Chetty U, Donnan P T, Forrest P, Hepburn W, Huggins A, Kirkpatrick A E, Lamb J, Muir B B and Prescott R J (1990), Edinburgh trial of screening for breast cancer: mortality at seven years, *Lancet*, February, 335, 241–6.

Roberts M M, French K and Duffy J (1984), Breast cancer and breast self-examination: what do Scottish women know?, *Social Science and Medicine*, 18, 791–7.

Rutter D R and Calnan M (1987), Do health beliefs predict health behaviour? A further analysis of breast self-examination. In H R Dent (Ed.) *Clinical Psychology: Research and Development*, London: Croom Helm.

Rutter D R, Calnan M, Vaile M S B, Field S and Wade K A (1992), Discomfort and pain during mammography: description, prediction and prevention, *British Medical Journal*, 305, 443–5.

Samuel E, Forrest A P M, Anderson T J, Fulton P M, Lutz W, Brough C, Loudon N B, Forbes W and Scott A M (1978), Screening for breast cancer (Report from Edinburgh Breast Screening Clinic), *British Medical Journal*, 2, 175–8.

Shapiro S (1977), Evidence on screening for breast cancer from a randomized trial, *Cancer*, 39, 2772–82.

Skrabanek P (1988), The debate over mass mammography in Britain – the case against, *British Medical Journal*, 297, 971–2.

Spielberger C D, Gorsuch R C and Lushene R E (1970), *Manual for the State-Trait Anxiety Inventory*, Palo Alto, Calif: Consulting Psychologists Press.

Stillman M (1977), Women's health beliefs about breast cancer and breast self-examination, *Nursing Research*, 26, 121.

Stomper P C, Kopans D B, Sadowsky N L, Sonnenfeld M R, Swann C A, Gelman R S, Meyer J E, Jochelson M S, Hunt M S and Allen P D (1988), Is mammography painful?, *Archives of International Medicine*, 148, 521–4.

Tabar L, Fagerberg G, Duffy S W and Day N E (1989), The Swedish two county trial of mammographic screening for breast cancer: recent results and calculation of benefit, *Journal of Epidemiology and Community Health*, 43, 107–14.

Tabar L, Fagerberg C J G, Gad A, Baldetorp L, Holmberg L H, Grontoft O, Ljungquist U, Lundstrom B and Manson J C (1985), Reduction in mortality from breast cancer after mass screening with mammography (Randomized trial from the Breast Cancer Screening Working Group of the Swedish National Board of Health and Welfare), *Lancet*, 13 April, 829–32.

Tsechkovski M, Semiglason V, Sagaidask V, Moiseyenko V and Mikhailov E (1986), Role of breast self-examination in reduction of mortality from breast cancer, Protocol of Study, Geneva, WHO.

UK Trial of Early Detection of Breast Cancer Group (1988), First results of mortality reduction in the UK trial of early detection of breast cancer, *Lancet*, 20 August, 411–16.

Vaile M S B, Calnan M, Rutter D R and Wall B (1993), Breast cancer screening services in three areas: uptake and satisfaction, *Journal of Public Health Medicine*, in press.

Verbeek A L M Holland R, Sturmans F, Hendriks J H C L, Mravunac M and Day N E (1984), Reduction of breast cancer mortality through mass screening with modern mammography, *Lancet*, June.

Vessey M (1991), *Breast Cancer Screening 1991: Evidence and Experience Since the Forrest Report*, Sheffield: NHSPSP Publications.

Warren R (1988), The debate over mass mammography in Britain – the case for, *British Medical Journal*, 297, 969–70.

Wright C J (1986), Breast cancer screening: a different look at the evidence, *Surgery*, 100, 4, 594–8.

Chapter 4

Motorcycling

In 1990, the most recent year for which official statistics are available, 659 motorcycle[1] riders and passengers were killed in Great Britain. The number seriously injured was 10,462, against 26,749 for car occupants, yet the number of cars registered in Great Britain was almost 24 times the number of motorcycles. When average distance travelled is taken into account, motorcyclists were more than six times more likely than car drivers to be involved in an injury accident, 18 times more likely to be injured themselves, and 35 times more likely to be killed or seriously injured. In collisions between a motorcycle and a car, the probability of death or serious injury was almost 35 times greater for those on the motorcycle than for those in the car. Almost 60 per cent of motorcycling accidents involved riders aged 24 or under, and the peak age for dying on a motorcycle was 17–19. Apart from injuries from other causes, only suicide and cancer claim more lives in the 15–24 age group (Department of Transport 1991; Office of Population Censuses and Surveys, 1991). The main purpose of this chapter is to identify the principal social inputs for accident involvement and to trace the paths of mediation between inputs and outcomes.

There are four sections. The first examines the accident statistics in detail. The second presents the existing social psychological literature on social inputs, behavioural outcomes

1. Throughout the chapter, 'motorcycle' includes all two-wheeled motor-driven vehicles.

and mediators. The third section of the chapter outlines our own programme of research, in which beliefs and attitudes about safe riding are being used to predict behaviour and accident liability. In the concluding section, we discuss the implications of our findings for theory, policy and practice.

Death and injury among motorcyclists

Every year, more than 5,000 people are killed on the roads of Great Britain. From the post-war peak of almost 8,000 a year in the mid-1960s, the figure has declined steadily to reach 5,217 in 1990 (Figure 4.1). When the number of deaths is expressed as a ratio against the population of the country, Britain has the 'safest roads' in the European Community, even allowing for the relatively large number of vehicles per capita, and also compares favourably with countries outside the EC.

When we turn to motorcyclists, the picture is even more encouraging, at first glance. Figure 4.2 gives the number of

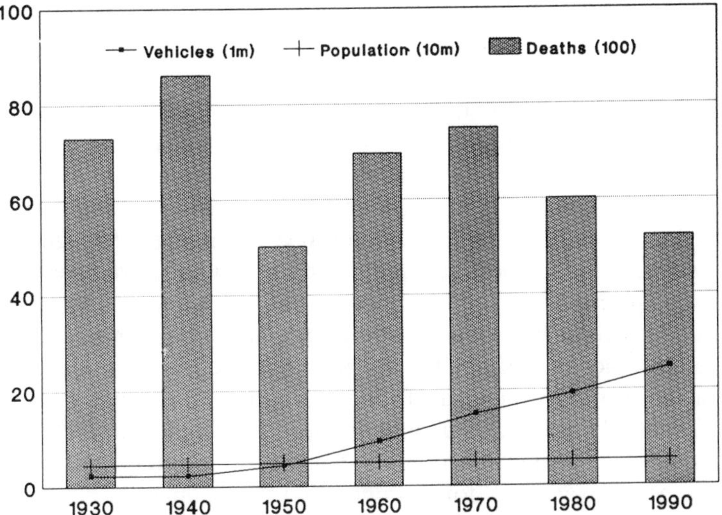

Figure 4.1 Road casualties: historical data. Source: Department of Transport

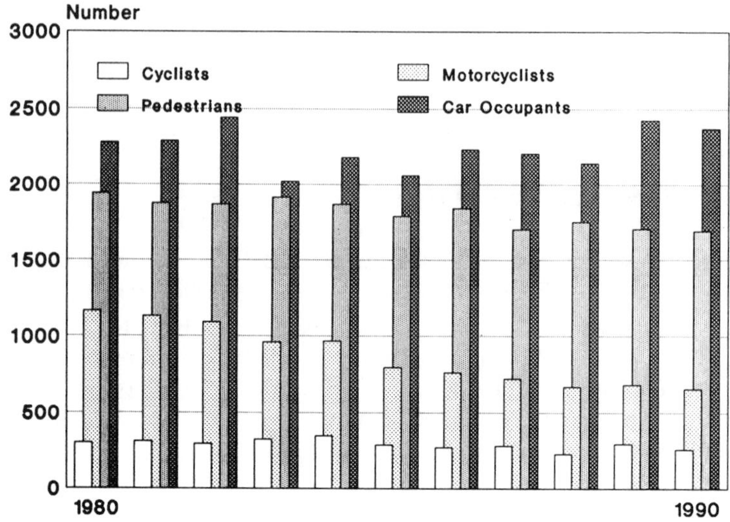

Figure 4.2 Number of deaths. Source: Department of Transport

deaths for the years 1980–90 by road user type. Car drivers and passengers were the largest group, followed by pedestrians, motorcyclists and their passengers, and then cyclists. Motorcyclists were the only group to show any significant change over the period, from 1,163 to 659 – a decline from 19 per cent of road deaths in 1980 to 13 per cent in 1990. The statistics for serious injuries – 21,543 in 1980 against 10,462 in 1990 – show a similar decline, though the figure for motorcyclists is high throughout. The reason is that very few motorcycling accidents produce only *minor* injuries.

Crude frequencies and distributions are misleading because they take account of neither the number of vehicles on the roads nor the distances they travel. There are, however, other ways of analyzing the data, and now the pattern and implications change dramatically. When the ratio of deaths to registered vehicles of all types is examined, for example, two things emerge. First, the ratios decline – from around 3,000 deaths per million vehicles in 1930 to just over 210 in 1990. But, second, the relative position of motorcyclists deteriorates. From 1930 to 1990, motorcycles fell from 31 per cent of registered vehicles to just over 3 per cent, but motorcyclist deaths fell by much less, from 25 per cent to 13 per cent of all road deaths – that is, from a little less than the 'pro rata' share to more than three times greater than pro rata. Moreover, while the 1950s onwards have seen a marked and continuing improvement in the ratio for vehicles overall, there has been no improvement at all for motorcyclists. The ratio of deaths to registered vehicles has always been greater for motorcycles than for vehicles overall, but it has become greater still in the last thirty or forty years.

A second way of breaking down the crude frequency data is to express casualties by vehicle kilometres – the number of registered vehicles in a category multiplied by the average distance they travel. In some respects, this produces the bleakest ratio of all for motorcyclists, for the figure is consistently high – twice as high as for cyclists, and twenty or thirty times as high as for car drivers, sometimes even higher (Figure 4.3). Government legislation has introduced many changes in the last fifteen years

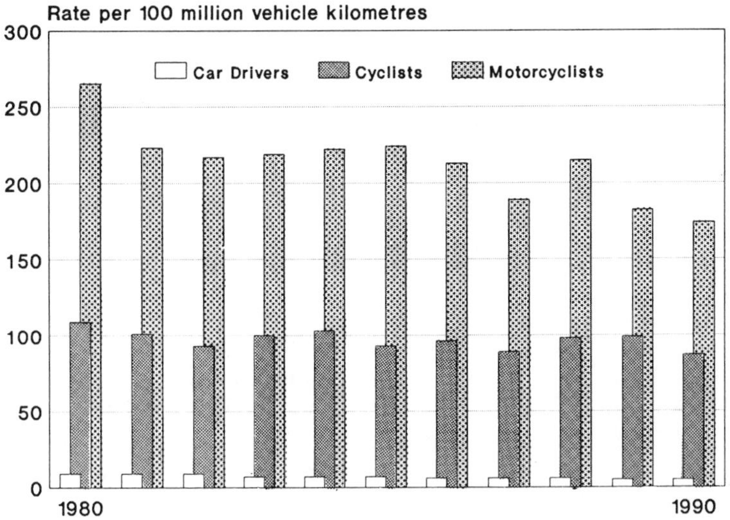

Figure 4.3 Death and serious injury rates. Source: Department of Transport

to try to reduce motorcycling accidents and their severity – compulsory safety helmets (1973) and improved design standards (1977 and 1980); stricter proficiency tests, and a reduction in the time a provisional licence can be held (1982); restrictions on engine capacity for learners (1983); and compulsory basic training (1990) – and it has spent large sums of money on education and publicity. While the number of motorcyclists has declined over the corresponding period, however, the casualty rate among those who remain has not.

Social inputs, behaviours and mediators

In this second section of the chapter, we examine the social psychological literature on inputs, behavioural outcomes and mediators, to try to find patterns in the casualty statistics we have just reviewed. The main inputs on which the literature has concentrated are age and training, and the main behaviours are wearing safety helmets and drink-riding. Unfortunately, little attempt has so far been made to link inputs to behavioural outcomes in any systematic way, but recent evidence has begun to point to the probable importance of perceived risk and attitudes. It was this recent work that provided the starting-point for our own research, to which we shall turn in the third section of the chapter.

Social inputs

Age of rider

The importance of age in accident involvement and outcome has been demonstrated many times, and published statistics from our own Department of Transport show the typical pattern. Almost 75 per cent of casualties in 1990 were to riders and passengers aged 29 or less, over 30 per cent to those aged 19 or less. The pattern is clearer still for casualty *rates* (Figure 4.4), where the number of riders in each group and the average distance they travel are taken into account. Car drivers show a similar trend, but both the peak and the decline in casualties with age are much less marked. What the published statistics do not show, of

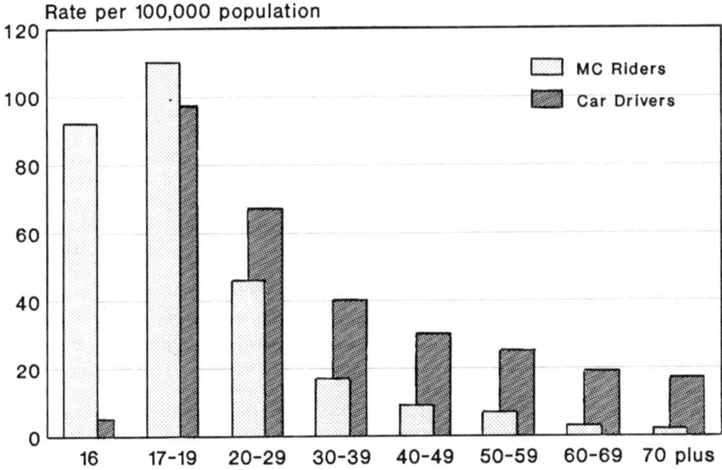

Figure 4.4 Casualty rates by age, 1990; deaths and serious injury. Note: the ratio of all registered vehicles to motorcycles is almost 30 : 1

course, is *how* age has its effects – the processes which link it to outcome – but a number of clues have begun to emerge from recent research on mediators, which we shall examine later.

Training

Statistics from the Department of Transport suggest that people who have received a formal training in motorcycling have worse accident records than those who have not. The possible relationship with age is difficult to disentangle – trained people are typically younger than those who are untrained because of the increased emphasis on training in recent years – but a number of studies in the United States have produced similar findings (for example, Jonah and Dawson, 1979; Jonah, Dawson and Bragg, 1981; Prem and Good, 1984).

One of the most important was by Mortimer (1984). The design was very simple and consisted of a comparison of riders who had taken a well-established course run by the American Motorcycle Safety Foundation with a group who had had no formal training. When age and years licensed were controlled, the group who had taken the course proved to be no better than the control group. In a further evaluation, Mortimer (1988) went on to compare 913 graduates of the course with a control group of 500 other riders on an extended selection of variables. Again, the findings showed little evidence that formal training was beneficial: 'those who had taken the course *did not* [our emphasis] have a lower violation rate, a lower accident rate, a lower total cost of damage to accident-involved motorcycles, a significantly lower mean cost of injury treatment per accident, or a lower total cost of injury treatment. Those who had taken the course *did* [our emphasis] have a lower mean cost of damage to the motorcycle per accident' (Mortimer, 1988, p. 187). As Mortimer had argued earlier: 'Attitudinal or personality variables may also be important in affecting the accident rate, since persons who indicated that they always used seat belts in automobiles had a lower accident rate when riding motorcycles. This may reflect . . . the possibility that such people do not take as many risks as others and are better able to estimate the actual risks involved in various tasks' (*ibid.*, p. 70). What mattered, for Mortimer, was mediators, and the likely candidate was perception of risks.

In a more recent paper, McDavid, Lohrmann and Lohrmann (1989) have suggested that the difficulty in finding positive effects of formal training may be an artifact of 'the lack of similarity between persons who seek motorcycle training and those who do not' (p. 62). McDavid and his colleagues stress the importance of matching experimental and control groups properly and assessing performance over a substantial time interval. Each formally trained rider in their sample was matched, therefore, with an untrained rider of the same age, sex and riding history (number of years' experience, number of previous accidents, and so on), and performance was assessed over a period of six years. The results showed that the untrained riders experienced 64 per cent more motorcycling accidents between 1979 and 1984 than those who were trained, and 32 per cent more than for *any* type of vehicle. Furthermore, in a discriminant analysis of 'all vehicle' accident involvement, it was found that formal motorcycle training was the second most significant predictor of (lack of) accidents. The first was age.

Behaviour

Wearing safety helmets

The benefits of wearing safety helmets began to be realized some fifty years ago (for example, Cairns, 1941; Cairns and Holbourn, 1943). It was only in 1973, however, that wearing a helmet became compulsory in Britain, several years after many US states had enacted their own legislation. Research on the benefits continued into the 1970s, often in the form of comparisons between states which *had* legislated and others which had not (for example, Kraus, Riggins and Franti, 1975a, 1975b; Robertson, 1976; Kraus *et al.*, 1976). Later, as a number of states deregulated, and removed compulsion, 'before' and 'after' changes became the focus (for example, National Highway Traffic Safety Administration, 1980; Watson, Zador and Wilks, 1981; Chenier and Evans, 1987). Consistently, helmets were found to save lives and minimize or even prevent injuries.

What most of the research did, however, was to ignore whether motorcyclists *wore* their helmets, but there were exceptions, two in particular. In the first, Williams, Ginsburg and Burchman (1979) compared two American states where helmets had remained compulsory for all riders (Maryland and Florida) with three states that had relaxed their legislation to allow riders over 18 years of age not to wear helmets (Louisiana, Arizona and Texas). There was a marked difference: 100 per cent of observed riders in Maryland and 98 per cent in Florida were observed wearing their helmets against only 39 per cent in Louisiana, 46 per cent in Arizona, and 63 per cent in Texas. Furthermore, almost half of riders estimated to be younger than 18 were without helmets in Louisiana and Arizona, even though in both states helmets were mandatory for that age group.

In the second paper, Simpson (1983) contested Williams, Ginsburg and Burchman (1979), for he found that riders who lived in American states without compulsory helmet laws (California and Colarado, Connecticut, Illinois, Indiana, Iowa, Maine, Rhode Island and Washington) still *reported* wearing helmets an average of almost 90 per cent of the time. Simpson's finding, however, was later questioned (by Simpson himself), for direct observation in two of the states revealed that only 48–68 per cent of riders *in fact* used their helmets, whatever they might have claimed – figures which were now consistent with those of

Williams, Ginsburg and Burchman. Riders who reported that they wore their helmets rarely or never, Simpson found, were less educated and younger than the others and tended to ride particular makes of machine. While 22 per cent of Harley-Davidson riders, for example, rarely or never wore a helmet, the figure for BMW riders was 2 per cent.

Drink-riding

It is estimated that around 20 per cent of people who are killed or seriously injured in road accidents in Great Britain are over the legal limit of 80 g of alcohol per 100 ml of blood, and the figure is probably an underestimate since samples are not taken from all victims. More than half of drink-related accidents involve no other vehicle, though many kill or injure a pedestrian. The overall figure for motorcyclists in 1990 was slightly lower than for drivers (18 per cent against 20 per cent), and the difference was particularly marked in the 30–39 age group.

Less extensive analyses from other countries have often reported that alcohol is relatively *unimportant* in motorcycling casualty statistics – for example, Raeder and Negri (1969) in the United States, Newman (1976) in Canada, and Vaughan (1976) in Australia. Baker and Fisher (1977), in contrast, found even higher rates of drink-riding in the United States than in Britain, in that an examination of 99 motorcyclists who were killed showed that 50 per cent were over the legal blood alcohol limit. Baker and Fisher point out, however, that no *causal* relationship can be established because we still lack reliable 'population' data on the prevalence of drink-riding – that is, among riders who do not have accidents as well as those who do. It is also possible, of course, that drinking and 'riding badly' both reflect some other factor, and it is this factor which 'causes' both – perhaps an underlying attitude, for example.

Mediators

Perceived risk

Early studies of 'subjective' or 'perceived' risk were concerned with car driving rather than motorcycle riding and they concentrated on the way drivers performed certain specific manoeuvres (for example, Cohen, Dearnaley and Hansel, 1958) or estimated the riskiness of particular situations (for example, Jones and Heimstra, 1964). As Colbourn (1978) pointed out, however, the data were seldom easy to interpret, even his own from computer simulations of 'gap-closure' tasks, for 'it may be expecting too much for drivers to express perceived risk overtly and accurately. Task variables, social pressures and expectancies, and experimenter effects may all interact with the subject's performance, producing a biased perception' (Colbourn, 1978, p. 140).

A methodology which avoids the need to report perceived risk overtly – but which again appears not to have been used with motorcyclists as yet – is field observation. Evans and Wasielewski (1981), for example, used time-recorded photographs to assess the 'headway' car drivers allowed between vehicles on a Canadian motorway. By referring registration numbers to the police, they were able to relate risk-taking to the driver's record of accidents and traffic law violations. The results showed that risk-taking was related both to number of accidents and to number of traffic violations. The study was part of a programme of research on Evans' 'human behaviour feedback' theory of road user behaviour (Evans, 1985, 1991).

In the literature on perception of risk by *motorcyclists*, rather less interest has been shown in *perceived* risk than *objective* risk – that is, actual probabilities. Nevertheless, a number of studies have attempted to relate estimates of risk to a variety of social inputs (for example, Knoflacher, 1974; Bragg, Dawson and Jonah, 1980; Bragg, 1981). According to Bragg, Dawson and Jonah (1980), for example, variables that contributed significantly to a discriminant analysis of accident-involved and accident-free motorcyclists included age, experience and marital status.

In a later study, in which perceived risk *was* addressed, Leaman and Fitch (1986) interviewed 72 British motorcyclists, and asked them to estimate the risk of having an accident and the risk of being killed in an accident 'in the next two years'. Generally, they underestimated the probability of an accident (range: 0–100 per cent; mean: 41 per cent) compared to their own past accident rates (mean: 0.74 per annum), but overestimated the risk of being killed (range: 0–70 per cent; mean: 16.3 per cent) compared to the national statistical probability (0.16 per cent). Furthermore, although perceived accident risk was unrelated to the rider's yearly accident rate or total number of accidents, it was significantly higher in riders who knew someone who had been involved in a serious accident than those who did not. Perceived fatality risk, in contrast, was directly related to the rider's own yearly accident rate and total number of accidents, as well as to knowledge of someone involved in a serious accident. Prior knowledge of a serious accident, Leaman and Fitch conclude, is the single most important factor in riders' perceptions of the risks of motorcycling.

In one final study of interest, Graham and Lee (1986) examined the way in which the concept of 'risk compensation' could be applied to effects of helmet legislation. According to the hypothesis of risk homeostasis/risk compensation (Adams, 1981, 1987; Wilde, 1982a, 1982b, 1985), when new safety measures are introduced, the human operator (in this case the rider) adjusts his or her behaviour to maintain all (in the case of the risk homeostasis hypothesis) or part (in the case of the risk compensation hypothesis) of a previous level of 'acceptable risk'. A real reduction in motorcycling accidents, it is argued, can be achieved only by changing the level of risk found acceptable by riders when operating their machines. What Graham and Lee suggested was that, although the introduction of compulsory helmet laws produces an immediate decline in motorcyclist mortality – and their repeal produces an immediate increase – there is 'also some evidence of gradual "risk compensation" behavior: The immediate rise in fatalities following repeal of helmet laws appears to dissipate gradually at a rate of roughly 2.5 percent per year' (Graham and Lee, 1986, p. 253).

Beliefs and attitudes

In the late 1980s, a new approach to mediators began to emerge, based on the attitude literature from social psychology, and it is to this new tradition that our own research belongs. The main questions are whether riders' beliefs and attitudes predict their behaviour and whether their behaviour predicts their liability to accidents. The attitude literature has already led to successful analyses of *drivers'* behaviour – notably wearing seat belts (Wittenbraker, Gibbs and Kahle, 1983; North and Spencer, 1984; Budd and Spencer, 1986; Nelson and Moffit, 1988; Sutton and Hallett, 1989; Stasson and Fishbein, 1990), using restraints and safety seats for children (Gielen *et al.*, 1984; Webb, Sanson-Fisher and Bowman, 1988) and drink-riding (Åberg *et al.*, 1991) – but few studies have yet been published on *motorcycling*. The most substantial so far is by Hobbs, Galer and Stroud (1983). Hobbs, Galer and Stroud derived their survey items from discussion groups, carried out in three British locations (Norwich in East Anglia, Greenock in Scotland, and London) selected according to relative accident rates and rainfall (a major factor in regional rates of ownership). From the variety of topics discussed by the groups, the authors were able to produce a list of attitudinal items concerning such things as 'maintenance/repairs/servicing', 'clothing', 'police', 'legislation', "training/education', 'other road users', 'accidents', and 'risk-taking'. The items were presented to subjects in the form of statements, with which they were asked to agree or disagree on five-point scales. The responses were then factor analyzed, and seven factors were identified, accounting for 85 per cent of the common variance: training, drivers, police, helmets, inherent pleasure, image and accident avoidance.

Although the factors were later used as the basis for a number of discriminant analyses, the original methodology was unfortunately such as to make any link between them and the accident liability of motorcyclists difficult to assess. A discriminant analysis carried out on 'experience of spills and accidents', for example, was able to relate riders' present attitudes to *past* accidents only, providing little evidence either for or against attitudes as *predictors* of accident involvement in the future. Furthermore, the study provided no systematic means by which attitudes could be related directly to behaviour. It is unclear, for example, given our discussion of the risk homeostasis hypothesis, whether attitudes such as 'wearing my helmet gives me a feeling of safety' will lead to *more* or *less* safe riding behaviour. Within the methodological framework used by Hobbs, Galer and Stroud it is impossible to say whether a positive (safety conscious) attitude would have any effect at all on the future behaviour of the person expressing it.

Implications from the literature review

An important conclusion to be drawn from the work we have examined – on social inputs, behavioural outcomes and mediators

– is that a *systematic* analysis is needed of the ways in which social psychological factors *mediate* social inputs and behavioural outcomes. Perceived risk is one important mediator, as we have shown. Research on riders' beliefs and attitudes, however, we believe has the most to offer, but progress has been slow. The main problem has been the lack of theoretical models, with the result that proper definition and measurement have been lacking and little attempt has been made to link attitudes directly to rider behaviour. In our own research, to which we now turn, the prediction of behaviour through theoretical models has been the main concern.

A programme of research

The purpose of our research has been to try to examine the ways in which social psychological variables *mediate* inputs and outcomes, where outcomes are riding behaviours and accidents. The particular mediators we have chosen to explore are riders' beliefs and attitudes which, as we have seen, the recent literature has begun to suggest *may* play a part in outcome. There are two problems in the published studies, however: first, no attempt has been made to examine the relationships systematically, by means of established theoretical models or accepted ways of conceptualizing beliefs and attitudes; and, second, none of the research has been prospective, which means that, since beliefs and behaviour have been measured at the same time, it is impossible either to make genuine *predictions* of behaviour or to avoid the contamination of beliefs by behaviour. The objectives of our own research have been threefold: to predict behaviour and accident involvement from beliefs and attitudes by means of a prospective design in which the principal dependent measures are behaviour and accident involvement in the twelve months *after* beliefs and attitudes have been measured; to use theoretical models to guide the structuring of our measures and analyses; and to arrive at a 'map' of mediation, in which the links between inputs and outcomes through beliefs and attitudes are shown diagrammatically as pathways. The theoretical models we have used are the Theory of Reasoned Action of Fishbein and Ajzen (1975) and its recent extension, the Theory of Planned Behaviour (Ajzen,

1988), and the Health Belief Model of Becker and his colleagues (Janz and Becker, 1984).

Theoretical models

Theory of Reasoned Action

The Theory of Reasoned Action provides a conceptual and empirical account of the relationships between beliefs, attitudes, intentions and behaviours, as we saw in Chapter 1. Behaviour which is under conscious control is underpinned by two sets of attitudes, Fishbein and Ajzen argue: our 'personal' attitude towards performing the behaviour or behaviours in question; and our 'subjective norm', which consists of our perceptions of how people who are important to us believe we ought to behave. Sometimes the two components will act together and reinforce each other, but sometimes they will be in opposition – the rider who 'personally' thinks that saving time is what matters but who knows his family think he should always obey the Highway Code. Each set of attitudes is underpinned in turn by a corresponding set of beliefs, which are the informational base of the model. From beliefs come attitudes, and from attitudes come intentions and so behaviour. The model offers a systematic analysis of specific beliefs and their consequent behaviours, and allows one to examine the social psychological factors that underpin safe and unsafe motorcycling and the individual and normative pressures that influence the degree of risk a rider finds acceptable.

Health Belief Model

The Health Belief Model takes a rather different view and provides a useful complement, as we saw in Chapter 1. It consists of three belief 'dimensions': perceived vulnerability, perceived severity and perceived benefits and barriers. Vulnerability in the present case is concerned with how likely motorcyclists believe they are to have accidents; severity is about the perceived seriousness of the consequences of accidents; and benefits and barriers are the perceived rewards and costs of the behaviours that help to prevent accidents. Benefits and barriers are reminiscent of Fishbein and Ajzen's behavioural beliefs, but the vulnerability and severity dimensions offer something quite different. The expectation is that people who ride 'safely' will be those who believe they are especially likely to have accidents, that the consequences will be severe, and that the benefits of riding safely outweigh the costs.

Recent work on the Health Belief Model has led to the inclusion of three additional factors, and these too we shall examine: locus of control; habit; and social support (King, 1982; Kristiansen, 1987). Locus of control describes people in terms of the extent to which they believe the outcomes of their behaviour are under their own 'internal' control, the 'external' control of other people and circumstances, or chance (Rotter, 1966). It is likely to be an important factor in explaining the behaviour of riders because the more we feel that other people, circumstances, or chance determine our behaviour, the less likely we are to take personal responsibility for our own safety. Encouraging riders to comply with safety regulations and recommendations as a matter of routine will be especially successful, the literature suggests, when the rider has strong social support (Langlie, 1977; Langer, 1978; Kristiansen, 1987) and compliance is learnt as a matter of 'family habit' (Allen and Taylor, 1984).

The investigation

Design, subjects and procedure

The main part of our programme of research has been a prospective postal survey of 4,101 motorcyclists sampled nationally. Riders' beliefs about safe riding were measured in the Spring of 1989 and were used to predict their behaviour twelve months later, along with their reports of accidents and spills in the intervening period. As part of an earlier survey by the Department of Transport, a random sample of 10,000 motorcycle keepers was taken from the central register at the then Driver Vehicle and Licensing Centre, and riders were asked to report and describe each of their accidents, if any, from February 1987 to February 1988. They were also asked whether they were willing to take part in further research, and a total of 4,777 agreed. The 4,777 formed the pool for our own research, and 4,101 were drawn at random for the present survey. Half the subjects were randomly assigned to receive a questionnaire based on the Theory of Reasoned Action (2,051), and half were assigned to receive one based on the Health Belief Model (2,050). The questionnaires had already been piloted (Rutter, Quine and Chesham, 1990, 1992), and they were sent out in their final form in April and May 1989 (Figure 4.5).

The questionnaire contained five sections: 'Safe riding', which examined beliefs (Tables 4.1 to 4.3) and locus of control (Table 4.4); 'You and your bike', covering the characteristics of the machine, the respondent's riding career, and current behaviour (Table 4.5); 'Spills and accidents', asking for details of mishaps

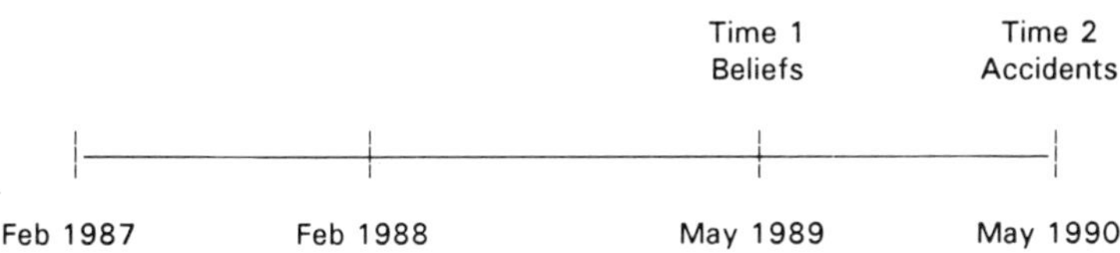

Figure 4.5 Design

Table 4.1 Reasoned Action behavioural belief items

BB 1	Being a safe rider means maintaining my bike properly
BB 2	Being a safe rider means not breaking the speed limit
BB 3	Being a safe rider means always wearing a crash helmet when riding
BB 4	Being a safe rider means not riding my bike after drinking alcohol
BB 5	Being a safe rider means obeying traffic laws
BB 6	Being a safe rider means using my headlamp during daylight
BB 7	Being a safe rider means doing what is taught on training courses
BB 8	Being a safe rider means following the Highway Code
BB 9	Being a safe rider means wearing bright or reflective clothing on my bike
BB 10	Being a safe rider means not riding too close behind other vehicles
BB 11	Being a safe rider means showing consideration for other road users
BB 12	Being a safe rider means concentrating properly when riding
BB 13	Being a safe rider means having crash bars on my bike

Table 4.2 Health Beliefs perceived vulnerability and severity items

Vulnerability
How likely do you think you are to have a serious accident needing hospital treatment in the next year compared with the following road users?

- Other motorcyclists
- Car drivers
- Pedal cyclists
- Pedestrians

Severity
If you had a serious accident in the next year needing hospital treatment, how seriously do you think it would affect your life?

- Your working life
- Your family life
- Your social life
- Your personal life

on the road in the preceding twelve months; 'Bikes and biking', a test of knowledge about riding and the road; and 'Some details about you', a set of demographic questions about age, education and occupation. The Reasoned Action and Health Belief versions differed only in the first section: the Reasoned Action questionnaire asked about belief strengths, outcome evaluations and normative beliefs,[2] while the Health Beliefs questionnaire asked about perceived vulnerability, perceived severity and benefits and barriers.

A year later, the Time 2 questionnaire was sent out, this time the same for both conditions. It asked about three things: current behaviour; spills and accidents since the Time 1 questionnaire; and 'exposure', which is an amalgam of measures about mileage, types of journey and types of road used most frequently designed

2. Because respondents would have differed in who were their salient referents, we asked only about the generalized 'people who are important to me'. No measure of 'motivation to comply' was taken since motivation to comply with a generalized referent makes little sense and would not have produced useful data.

Table 4.3 Health Beliefs benefit and barrier items

Maintaining your bike	.. makes it perform better
	.. takes time and expense
Breaking the speed limit	.. is fun
	.. risks having an accident
Wearing a crash helmet	.. gives you a feeling of being safe
	.. restricts vision
Riding after drinking alcohol	.. gives you increased confidence
	.. makes your reactions slower
Obeying the traffic laws	.. increases safety
	.. slows you down
Using your headlamp during daylight	.. helps people to see you better
	.. flattens your battery
Doining what is taught on training courses	.. gives you a sense of skill
	.. slows down travelling time
Following the Highway Code	.. makes you feel safe
	.. means others take advantage of you
Wearing bright or reflective clothing	.. helps people to see you better
	.. looks stupid
Riding too close behind other vehicles	.. makes overtaking easier
	.. risks having an accident
Showing consideration for other road users	.. earns you goodwill
	.. means they take advantage of you
Concentrating properly when riding	.. gives you a feeling of safety
	.. is tiring
Having crash bars on your bike	.. means less damage to your machine
	.. restricts handling

to provide an index of accident likelihood attributable simply to the type of riding done. Both the Time 1 and Time 2 questionnaires were made up as stapled A5 booklets, the first

Table 4.4 Locus of Control items

LC1	If I get into a dangerous situation on my bike I have the skill to get out of it safely
LC 2	Often I feel that no matter what I do, if I am going to have an accident it will just happen
LC 3	If I do what the Highway Code says, I am less likely to have accidents
LC 4	If I have an accident it's usually just chance
LC 5	I can only avoid accidents by doing what training experts advise
LC 6	Other road users play a big part in whether I have accidents or not
LC 7	If I get into a dangerous situation on my bike it's my own fault
LC 8	Obeying the law helps me avoid accidents
LC 9	If I get into a dangerous situation on my bike I just have to let things take their natural course
LC 10	Avoiding accidents is just plain luck
LC 11	If I have an accident I know it's because I haven't been taking proper care
LC 12	If I have an accident it's likely to be another road user's fault
LC 13	Even if I ride carefully it's easy to have an accident
LC 14	If I have an accident it's a matter of fate
LC 15	I can usually avoid accidents by riding carefully
LC 16	Following the Highway Code is the best way to avoid accidents
LC 17	I am directly responsible for my accidents
LC 18	Avoiding accidents depends on how well I ride

covering twenty sides, the second ten. Subjects were sent a covering letter from the Department of Transport, and the first page of the questionnaire outlined the purpose of the questions. A pre-paid business reply envelope was enclosed for respondents to return the questionnaire to us, and reminders were posted at three-weekly intervals to those who had not yet replied: a postcard after three weeks; a duplicate questionnaire at six weeks; and a second postcard at nine weeks. At Time 1, completed questionnaires were received from 64 per cent of respondents plus 7 per cent who were no longer riding, a total of 71 per cent. A year later, 62 per cent of subjects who had replied at Time 1 completed the Time 2 questionnaire, plus 24 per cent

Table 4.5 Behaviour items

Behaviour 1	Maintaining your bike
Behaviour 2	Breaking the speed limit on your bike
Behaviour 3	Wearing a crash helmet when riding
Behaviour 4	Riding your bike after drinking alcohol
Behaviour 5	Breaking the traffic laws on your bike
Behaviour 6	Using your headlamp during daylight
Behaviour 7	Doing what is taught on training courses
Behaviour 8	Breaking the Highway Code when riding
Behaviour 9	Wearing bright or reflective clothing on your bike
Behaviour 10	Riding too close behind another vehicle
Behaviour 11	Showing consideration for other road users
Behaviour 12	Losing your concentration when riding

who were no longer riding, a total of 86 per cent. Response rates for the Reasoned Action and Health Belief conditions were almost identical, at both Time 1 and Time 2.

The characteristics of the respondents, based on Time 1 information, were as follows. Men made up 87 per cent of the sample, and just over one third of respondents were under 30 years old while more than half were between 30 and 59. The age categories were chosen deliberately in our analysis to correspond to those used by insurance companies – whose main interest, of course, is accident involvement. More women than men, proportionately, were inexperienced motorcyclists, and there were differences too in educational attainments, the largest category of men having technical qualifications, the largest category of women having no formal qualifications at all. Only a minority of respondents had undergone formal motorcycling training, and older riders were the least likely, reflecting changes over the years in road safety practices and legislation, as we noted earlier in the chapter. Up to the age of 24, men were more likely than women to have been trained, but the pattern reversed from 25 onwards, probably because many of the older women had started riding only recently, when the move towards compulsory training had gained momentum.

The biggest sex difference was in size of machine: more than two-thirds of women were riding machines of no more than 50cc, while almost the same proportion of men were riding machines between 51cc and 500cc. Machine size for men was strongly age-related, but the predominance of 50cc machines for women held for all age groups. Government legislation prohibits machines over 125cc for people who have not yet passed their official proficiency test, and the implication is that men graduate to larger machines as soon as possible but the majority of women do not.

Accidents and behaviour at Time 1

Table 4.6 presents our findings for accident involvement in the twelve months to Time 1, broken down by demographic and other information. Young, inexperienced, trained riders were more likely to report accidents than those who were older, more experienced and untrained, while riders with formal educational qualifications were more likely to have had accidents than those without – probably reflecting age and experience and perhaps training too. There were no effects for sex of rider or size of machine. The pattern for age was even clearer when narrower bands were used – especially for men, for whom a steep decrease was evident from 17 to 60 plus.

The important question, of course, is whether accident history is related to behaviour. Mean values for the twelve behaviours and their relationship with accident history are shown in Table 4.7. For eight of the behaviours a significant effect emerged, and the most reliable were that riders who reported accidents had speeded more frequently than other riders, had more often broken traffic laws and the Highway Code, and had more frequently ridden too close behind other road users. Principal components analysis confirmed that the four behaviours belonged together, in a factor we labelled 'Breaking Law and Rules'. Breaking Law and Rules was the first factor to emerge in the analysis (Eigen value 2.9) – followed by 'Taking Care' (1.9), 'Carelessness' (1.1), and 'Safety Equipment and Training' (1.0) – and both for that reason and because of the strength of its relationship with accident history, it will provide the focus for much of our later discussion. When the pattern was re-examined by discriminant analysis, which controls for the interrelatedness between behaviours, speeding again emerged first.

Earlier, we saw that young men were the most likely to have accidents, and the remaining question for this section is whether the behaviour of young men differed from the behaviour of other

Table 4.6 Accidents in twelve months to Time 1

		% reporting accident	Chi^2
Age	Up to 19	29.3	83.5 ***
	20–29	18.7	
	30–59	10.5	
	60 plus	6.4	
Sex	Male	14.3	0.4
	Female	13.0	
Experience	Up to 2 years	29.5	93.3 ***
	3 years	26.1	
	4 years	23.5	
	5–9 years	15.1	
	10 years plus	9.9	
Training	Trained	20.3	23.8 ***
	Untrained	12.3	
Education	No qualifications	9.2	36.6 ***
	Up to O level	19.9	
	A level	16.8	
	Technical	12.0	
	Degree	19.7	
Machine Size	Up to 125cc	14.9	1.3
	126–500cc	13.8	
	501cc plus	13.0	

N = 2537, of whom 358 (14.1%) reported one or more accidents or spills.
*** $p < 0.001$

people. The answer is that it did, and the pattern is especially clear for Breaking Law and Rules: for speeding, breaking traffic laws and the Highway Code, and riding too close behind other road users, the values rose until the mid-twenties and then fell. For all four measures, the trends were highly significant statistically.

Beliefs and behaviour at Time 1

The main purpose of our analysis at Time 1 was to trace the paths of mediation from 'social inputs' to 'outcome', in this case

Table 4.7 Accidents in twelve months to Time 1 by behaviour

	Accidents		No accidents		
	Mean	SD	Mean	SD	t
Maintenance	3.6	1.1	3.6	1.1	0.0
Speeding	2.9	1.3	2.4	1.3	6.9 ***
Wearing helmet	4.9	0.5	4.9	0.7	1.0
Drink-riding	1.3	0.7	1.2	0.6	1.3
Breaking traffic laws	2.3	1.1	2.0	1.0	6.3 ***
Using daytime headlamp	3.6	1.5	3.3	1.6	3.1 ***
Doing as taught	3.1	1.4	3.2	1.4	1.7
Breaking Highway Code	2.4	1.0	2.1	1.0	6.3 ***
Wearing bright clothing	2.5	1.6	2.7	1.6	2.0 *
Riding too close	2.1	0.9	1.8	0.9	5.0 ***
Showing consideration	4.0	0.8	4.1	0.8	3.1 **
Losing concentration	2.0	0.9	1.8	0.8	3.6 ***

* $p < 0.05$
** $p < 0.01$
*** $p < 0.001$

behaviour. As we said in the previous section, we shall concentrate on the factor 'Breaking Law and Rules'. In general, we shall focus on men, because they made up almost 90 per cent of the sample, and we shall often break down the data by age because of the association with accident involvement we have seen already.

The starting-point for our analyses was locus of control, which was measured in both the Reasoned Action and Health Beliefs versions of the questionnaire. The items were first examined by principal components analysis, and four factors emerged: Chance, Powerful Others, Internal – as in traditional analyses of the Multidimensional Health Locus of Control scale – and one other, which we labelled 'My Skill/Others' Mistakes'. Men generally attributed their accident involvement and avoidance less to chance than to the other factors, but there were noticeable effects of age. From the age of 25, both Internal and Powerful Others rose while Chance fell slightly from its peak at 18–24, so that men in the age group most likely to have accidents saw accident involvement as more a matter of chance than did men who were older, and less a matter of either their own or others' behaviour. The effects of age were particularly strong for Powerful Others but for the fourth factor, My Skill/Others' Mistakes, there was no clear pattern.

Reasoned Action analysis. The core of the Reasoned Action model is behavioural and normative beliefs. Principal components analysis of the twelve behavioural belief items revealed four factors, which we labelled 'Obeying Law and Rules', 'Taking Care', 'Safety Equipment and Training' and 'Avoiding Risks'. The first, which corresponded to the first factor for behaviour, accounted for more variance than the other three factors combined, and there were noticeable effects of age, particularly an increase in law-abiding beliefs from the age of 25 – the age from which Breaking Law and Rules *behaviour* declined. The principal components analysis for normative beliefs revealed two factors, 'Taking Care' and 'Safety Equipment and Training'. Again the first factor was very strong, and again there were marked effects of age, in general indicating an increase in perceived social pressure to behave 'properly' from the age of 25 onwards.

The task now was to trace the paths of mediation from social inputs to behavioural outcome, and our first approach was to build a 'theoretical' hierarchical model. The purpose of the model was to order the variables in blocks in such a way that the order made sense as a causal chain. After that, two types of analysis would be conducted: hierarchical regression, which tests whether each block makes a significant additional contribution to outcome beyond that made by the accumulated previous blocks; and path analysis, which breaks down the blocks into their components and examines the direct and indirect links between individual variables.

The hierarchical model we developed for the Reasoned Action analysis is shown in Figure 4.6. The first mediating block, we argued, would be locus of control and perceived risk, which are sometimes seen as personality indices, so fundamental and pervasive are their presumed role in people's attributions about causality. Next came the Reasoned Action variables, behavioural and normative beliefs, which we placed alongside each other at

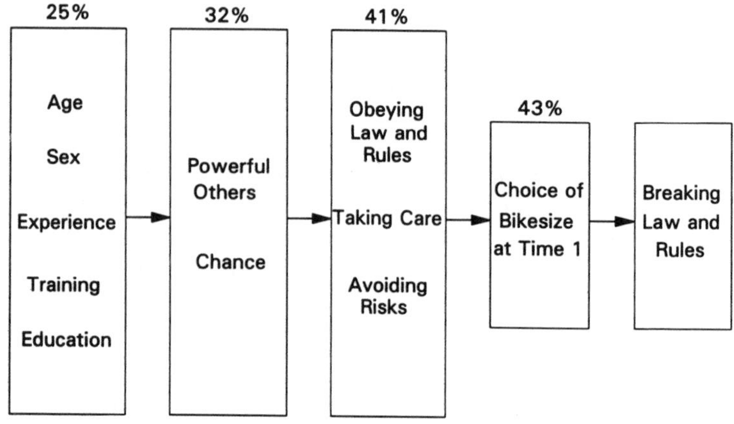

Figure 4.6 Reasoned action: hierarchical analysis for Time 1. Includes all variables that made a significant contribution to the path analysis at $p < 0.01$. Obeying Law and Rules, Taking Care, and Avoiding Risks are all behavioural beliefs factors

one level, as Fishbein and Ajzen prescribe. Finally came size of machine, which we regard as a *choice* because it is based in part on beliefs about safe riding: the bigger the machine, the greater the range of behaviours available to the rider.

The results of the hierarchical analysis are shown in Figure 4.6. Path analysis, which we shall report below, showed that a number of components made no contribution to outcome at the 1 per cent level of significance, and they were therefore dropped from the hierarchical analysis: 'Internal' and 'My Skill/Others' Mistakes' from locus of control, perceptions of risk, 'Safety Equipment and Training' from behavioural beliefs, and both the normative belief factors. What emerged from the remainder was that 43 per cent of the variance for Breaking Law and Rules was explained in total, and each of the blocks made a significant contribution to the explained variance in addition to that made already by the preceding blocks. The empirical results thus supported our *theoretical* ordering of variables and confirmed that the variables of interest to us acted as *mediators* between inputs and outcomes.

Hierarchical analysis is concerned with 'blocks' of variables, and does not allow one to identify the *individual* variables through which the relationships between inputs and outcomes are mediated. For that, we turned to path analysis. As we have seen in Chapters 2 and 3, path analysis consists of a series of multiple regression analyses, which attempt to predict each variable from every other, according to one's hypothesized model. The result is a map of mediating paths in which both direct and indirect paths from inputs to outcomes are shown, along with the strengths of the relationships in the form of beta weights.

The path analysis for Breaking Law and Rules is shown in Figure 4.7, and three main points emerge. First, each of the five inputs *did* lead to behaviour, sometimes directly but always by mediation. Age, for example, had a direct effect on behaviour, which could not be explained by mediation, but it also led to Powerful Others, to belief in Obeying Law and Rules, and to Choice of Bikesize, all of which in turn led eventually to

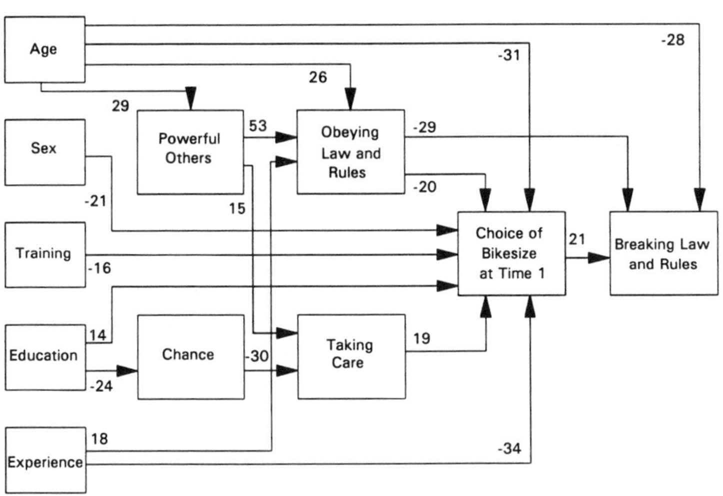

Figure 4.7 Reasoned action: path analysis for Time 1. Variables with incomplete paths or with betas below 0.125 are not shown. Decimal points for beta weights are omitted. Obeying Law and Rules and Taking Care are behavioural belief factors

behaviour. In other words, much of the effect of age on behaviour was due to its effects on perceptions, attributions and beliefs. The second point to emerge was that both locus of control (in the form of Powerful Others and Chance) and beliefs played an important part. Behavioural beliefs ('Obeying Law and Rules') and normative beliefs ('Taking Care') were both represented, emphasizing the importance of separating the two in the way the Theory of Reasoned Action suggests. The third point to note is that Choice of Bikesize was pivotal: there were direct paths from seven of the nine preceding variables, and it went on to play a significant part in behaviour.

As was to be expected from the univariate analyses, age proved to be particularly interesting. The older the rider, the less he or she reported breaking the law and rules (direct effect, beta −0.28), and the smaller the machine he or she chose to ride (−0.31), probably because of the large number of 'middle-aged' commuters. Older riders were more likely than younger riders to see their accident involvement and avoidance as in part attributable to other people (0.29 with Powerful Others), and they were more likely to believe in obeying the law and rules (0.26). Powerful Others and Obeying Law and Rules were themselves strongly related (0.53). Belief in obeying the law and rules was related negatively to both Choice of Bikesize (−0.20) and behaviour (−0.29), and Choice of Bikesize itself was related positively to behaviour (0.21), as we have seen already. Powerful Others led also to the normative belief, 'Taking Care' (0.15), which in turn was related positively to Choice of Bikesize (0.19), and so to behaviour.

A similar tracing of paths can, of course, be done for all the other social inputs – sex, training, education and experience – and the result is a detailed map which other techniques of analysis are unable to reveal. To re-emphasize the main conclusions: social inputs *were* related to behaviour, both directly and indirectly; locus of control, behavioural beliefs and normative beliefs all played a significant part in mediating the relationships; and the choice of machine size was pivotal.

Health Beliefs analysis. The distinctive features of the Health Belief Model are perceived vulnerability, perceived severity, and perceived benefits and barriers. Perceived vulnerability and severity were both made up of four items, which were scored from 1 to 5. Cronbach's alphas were 0.61 for vulnerability and 0.80 for severity, and items were therefore averaged to give scale scores. Principal components analysis of perceived benefits revealed four factors, which we labelled 'Feeling Safe', 'Being Seen', 'Having Fun' and 'Good Bike Performance and Safety'. For perceived barriers there were five factors: 'Others Take Advantage', 'Time', 'Restricted Handling', 'Risk of Accident' and 'Poor Human Performance and Safety'.

As in the Reasoned Action analysis, there were many effects for age. Perceived vulnerability revealed one, a belief among riders aged 18–24 that they were more at risk of an accident than other motorcyclists – which, of course, is accurate, according to the published statistics. For perceived severity, three of the four items produced a significant pattern and, in each case, there was a peak during the years when the rider was likely to have the responsibility of a family – again an accurate assessment. For perceived benefits there were many significant effects but no readily detectable pattern, and for perceived barriers there were rather fewer effects and again no clear pattern.

The next stage was to set up and test a hierarchical model, as we had done with the Reasoned Action data. Perceived vulnerability and severity were placed at the same level as locus of control (Figure 4.8), leaving perceived benefits and barriers to take up the next level, in the same position as behavioural and normative beliefs in the Reasoned Action model. Again there was good support for our theoretical position. A total of 44 per cent of the variance for Breaking Law and Rules was explained (against 43 per cent in the Reasoned Action analysis), and the three mediating blocks each added significantly to the variance explained by the accumulated preceding blocks – rather more, in fact, than was the case with the Reasoned Action model.

The final stage was to produce a path analysis as before, and the results are shown in Figure 4.9. There are four main points to make. First, the only factor from locus of control to act as a mediator was Powerful Others. Second, perceived vulnerability and severity, which were placed in the model at the same level as locus of control, played no part. Third, perceived benefits and barriers, represented by 'Having Fun' for benefits and 'Risk of Accident' for barriers, were each linked to behaviour through two paths: directly; and indirectly through Choice of Bikesize.

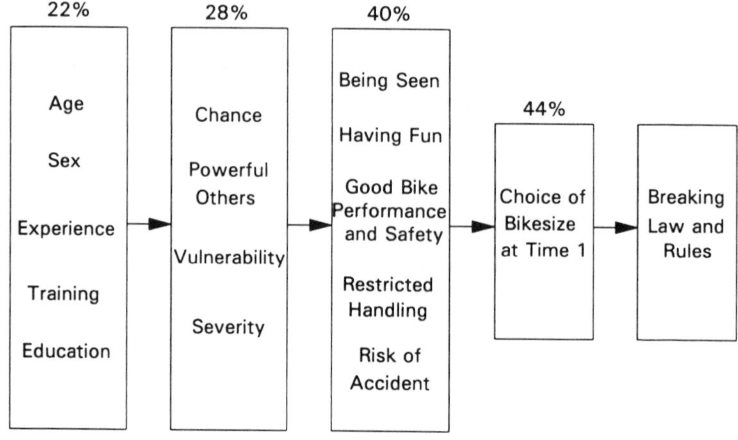

Figure 4.8 Health beliefs: hierarchical analysis for Time 1. Includes all variables that made a significant contribution to the path analysis at $p < 0.01$. Being Seen to Risk of Accident are benefit and barrier factors

Fourth, Choice of Bikesize was once again pivotal, since every preceding variable except Powerful Others had a direct path to it, and it went on in turn to have a significant influence on behaviour.

The net effect is a path diagram very similar to that for the Reasoned Action analysis, which reaffirms the role of perceptions, attributions and beliefs as mediators between social inputs and behavioural outcomes. Overall, it appeared to make little difference whether beliefs were conceptualized and measured according to the Theory of Reasoned Action or the Health Belief Model. It is noticeable, however, that the only distinctive components of the Health Belief Model to appear in the diagram were perceived benefits and barriers, for perceived vulnerability and severity played no part. Perceived benefits and barriers are concerned with the expected consequences of particular behaviours, and their positive or negative weightings. They therefore closely resemble the expectancy-value conception of behavioural outcomes, the theoretical basis of behavioural and normative beliefs in the Theory of Reasoned Action.

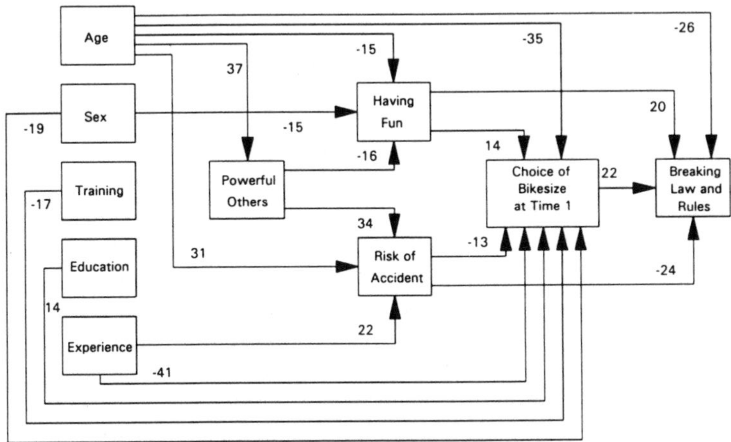

Figure 4.9 Health beliefs: path analysis for Time 1. Variables with incomplete paths and/or betas below 0.125 are not shown. Decimal points for beta weights are omitted. Having Fun is a benefit factor and Risk of Accident is a barrier factor

Accidents and behaviour at Time 2

In the twelve months to Time 2, 13.6 per cent of the sample had at least one spill or accident, compared with 14.1 per cent in the twelve months to Time 1. Of those who had reported an accident at Time 1, 30 per cent reported at least one more in the next twelve months, while 89 per cent of those who were accident-free at Time 1 continued to be accident-free at Time 2. Social inputs, it emerged, were related to accident involvement in almost exactly the same way as at Time 1, so that age, experience, training and education *were* associated with accident involvement, while sex of rider and size of machine were not. The measures of exposure we introduced at Time 2 also proved to be significant sources of variance, for accident involvement was related to high mileage, high frequency of trips and winter riding, as might be expected, but not to type of roads used most frequently. An additional finding was that riders who drove cars more than 5,000 miles a year were relatively 'protected' against accidents when riding. The pattern may, perhaps, be confounded with age and experience, but it may also suggest that riding and driving share a common underpinning, which is strengthened by either type of road experience.

From social inputs and exposure we turned next to behaviour, and the overwhelming pattern we found was one of consistency from Time 1 to Time 2 (Table 4.8): strong correlations for each of the twelve behaviours, and small but consistent changes in particular behaviours. Speeding, for example, showed a correlation of 0.74 between Time 1 and Time 2, but also a barely perceptible increase in mean values from 2.5 to 2.6 – which, because it was consistent across individuals, produced a highly significant t-value of 4.0. The implication is that most of what we examined was habitual by Time 2, but minor changes nevertheless occurred, and in the same direction from person to person.

The next question was whether behaviour would predict

Table 4.8 Behaviour at Time 1 and Time 2

	Time 1		Time 2			
	Mean	SD	Mean	SD	r	t
Maintenance	3.7	1.0	4.0	0.9	0.51 ***	13.0 ***
Speeding	2.5	1.3	2.6	1.2	0.74 ***	4.0 ***
Wearing helmet	4.9	0.5	5.0	0.3	0.11 ***	3.1 **
Drink-riding	1.2	0.6	1.3	0.6	0.42 **	2.6 **
Breaking traffic laws	2.0	1.0	2.1	1.1	0.54 ***	2.7 **
Using daytime headlamp	3.3	1.6	3.5	1.2	0.71 ***	7.0 ***
Doing as taught	3.4	1.3	3.8	1.1	0.46 ***	8.9 ***
Breaking Highway Code	2.1	0.9	2.2	0.9	0.48 ***	2.3 *
Wearing bright clothing	2.7	1.6	2.7	1.5	0.66 ***	0.3
Riding too close	1.9	0.9	2.0	0.9	0.46 ***	4.8 ***
Showing consideration	4.2	0.7	4.3	0.7	0.38 ***	7.0 ***
Losing concentration	1.8	0.8	1.8	0.8	0.39 ***	0.7

* $p < 0.05$
** $p < 0.01$
*** $p < 0.001$

accident involvement, and the short answer is that it did. Table 4.9 shows Time 2 accident involvement in relation to Time 2 behaviours and Time 1 behaviours. In both cases, speeding, breaking traffic laws, riding too close and losing concentration were the leading predictors. The pattern was generally similar to that for Time 1 accidents, and it is interesting to note that Time 2 accident involvement was predicted just as well by Time 1 behaviours as by Time 2 behaviours. Again, the implication is that habit plays an important part.

Patterns of mediation for accidents at Time 2

The final stage of our analysis was to map the patterns of mediation between social inputs and behavioural outcome at Time 2. As at Time 1, the first technique we used was hierarchical regression, and the hierarchical models we tested are shown in Figure 4.10 for the Reasoned Action analysis and Figure 4.11 for the Health Beliefs analysis. Again we confined ourselves to Law and Rule Breaking, and there were two levels

Table 4.9 Accidents in twelve months to Time 2 by mean behaviour

	Time 1 Behaviour			Time 2 Behaviour		
	Accidents	No accidents	t	Accidents	No accidents	t
Maintenance	3.7	3.7	0.7	4.0	4.0	0.1
Speeding	2.8	2.4	4.0 ***	2.9	2.5	4.4 ***
Wearing helmet	5.0	4.9	1.3	5.0	5.0	0.1
Drink-riding	1.3	1.2	1.0	1.3	1.2	0.6
Breaking traffic laws	2.3	2.0	3.8 ***	2.4	2.0	4.3 ***
Using daytime headlamp	3.5	3.3	1.9	3.7	3.5	2.2 *
Doing as taught	3.3	3.4	0.3	3.8	3.8	0.5
Breaking Highway code	2.3	2.1	3.1 **	2.3	2.1	2.0
Wearing bright clothing	2.7	2.8	0.7	2.6	2.8	1.7
Riding too close	2.1	1.8	4.5 ***	2.1	1.9	2.7 **
Showing consideration	4.1	4.2	0.6	4.2	4.3	1.3
Losing concentration	1.9	1.8	2.6 **	2.0	1.8	2.8 **

* $p < 0.05$
** $p < 0.01$
*** $p < 0.001$

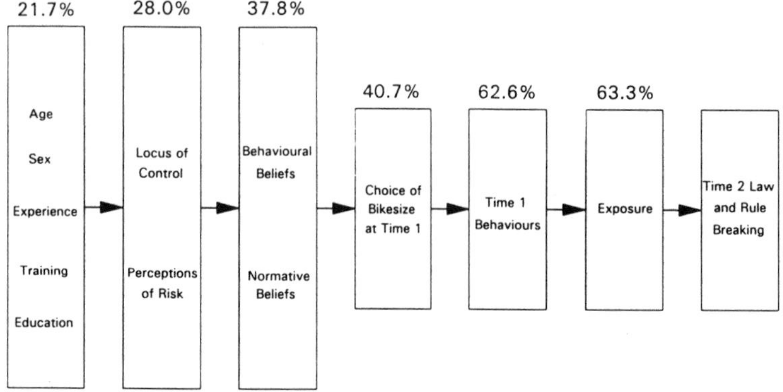

Figure 4.10 Reasoned action: hierarchical analysis for Time 2. Each level adds significantly to the variance accumulated by the preceding levels – except Exposure

to add to those we examined at Time 1 – Time 1 behaviours and exposure. The Time 1 behaviours were factor scores for Breaking Law and Rules and the other three factors that had emerged, namely Taking Care, Carelessness and Safety Equipment and Training; the exposure measures were annual mileage, number of trips per week, road types, seasons and annual car mileage.

Two main findings emerged: each level in the hierarchy added significantly to the variance accumulated by the preceding levels, with the exception of exposure in the Reasoned Action analysis; and the final variance explained was 63.3 per cent for the Reasoned Action analysis and 62.0 per cent for the Health Beliefs analysis. Behavioural beliefs and normative beliefs added a little under 10 per cent to the variance in the Reasoned Action analysis, and perceived benefits and barriers added a little over 10 per cent in the Health Beliefs analysis. The greatest increment in both cases came from Time 1 behaviour – over 20 per cent in the Reasoned Action analysis and 12 per cent in the Health Beliefs analysis. Thus, social inputs and behavioural outcomes *were* mediated by beliefs, previous behaviour and exposure, in the way our hierarchical models proposed; the final proportions of variance explained were large; and, as at Time 1, there was

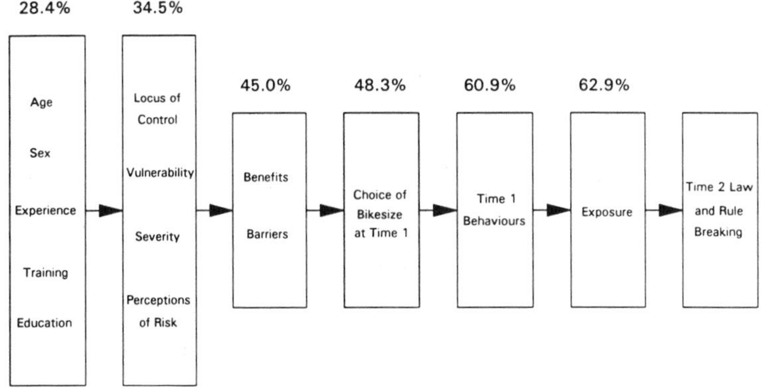

Figure 4.11 Health beliefs: hierarchical analysis for Time 2. Each level adds significantly to the variance accumulated by the preceding levels

little to choose between the Reasoned Action approach and the Health Beliefs approach.

The other technique of analysis we used was path analysis once again, and the first thing to say is that both the Reasoned Action and Health Beliefs data produced much more complex patterns at Time 2 than at Time 1. The analysis for the Reasoned Action data is shown in Figure 4.12, and there are several points to highlight. First, the five demographic inputs all led through mediation to behavioural outcome. From age, for example, there were direct paths to Powerful Others (locus of control), to Obeying Law/Rules and Safety Equipment/Training (behavioural beliefs), to Choice of Bikesize at Time 1, and to Time 1 Breaking Law/Rules (behaviour). All the paths led directly or through further mediation to outcome. Second, while the only effects of locus of control were mediated by behavioural beliefs, both measures of perceived risk (which had played no part at Time 1) led directly to outcome, though the paths were relatively weak. Third, all four behavioural beliefs acted as mediators, but no part was played by normative beliefs. Fourth, Choice of Bikesize was pivotal, just as at Time 1, for a number of demographic inputs led directly to it, and in turn it went on directly and through

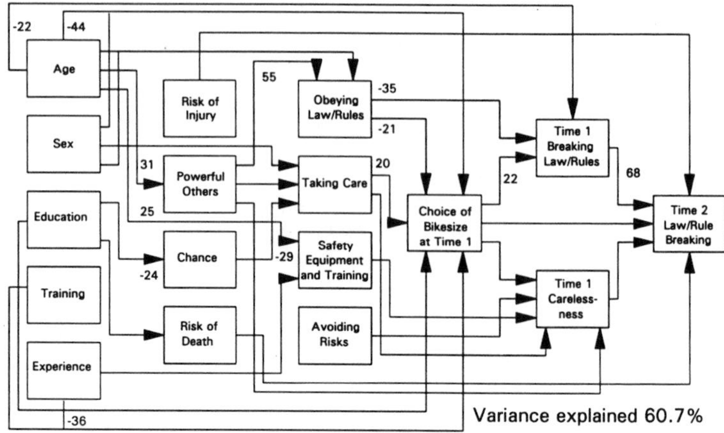

Figure 4.12 Reasoned action: path analysis for Time 2. Includes all variables with paths $p < 0.01$, but only those with betas 0.1 or greater are shown. Values are printed only for betas 0.2 or greater, and decimal points are omitted. Obeying Law and Rules to Avoiding Risks are all behavioural belief factors

mediation to outcome. Fifth, none of the indices of exposure played any part. Finally, the strongest predictor of outcome was the corresponding behaviour at Time 1, Breaking Law and Rules, an indication of the importance of habit. When Time 1 behaviour was removed from the analysis, the variance explained for Time 2 law and rule breaking fell to 38.4 per cent (Figure 4.13).

The analysis for the Health Beliefs data is shown in Figure 4.14, and the most important points to note are these. First, all five demographic inputs led to outcome, through mediation. Second, all the effects of locus of control, perceived vulnerability and severity, and perceived risk were mediated by perceived benefits and barriers – that is, there were no direct paths to later stages of the model. Third, Choice of Bikesize at Time 1 was pivotal, just as in the Reasoned Action analysis. Fourth, the only measure of exposure to be implicated was the number of trips each week, and the effect was small. Finally, the strongest predictor of outcome was once again Time 1 Breaking Law and

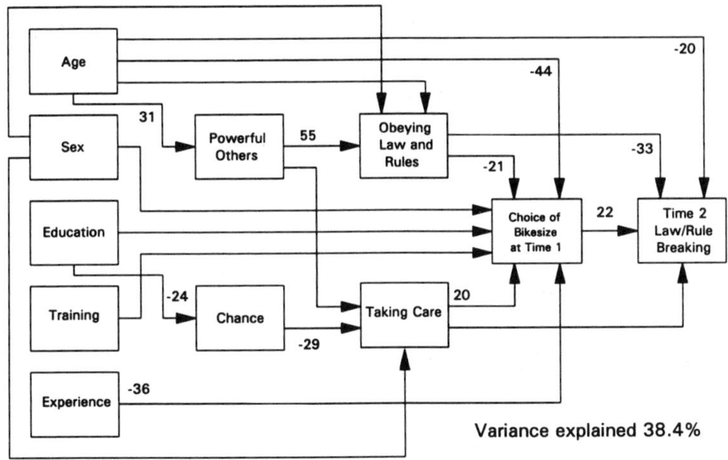

Figure 4.13 Reasoned action: Time 2 path analysis excluding prior behaviour. Includes all variables with paths $p < 0.01$, but only those with betas 0.1 or greater are shown. Values are printed only for betas 0.2 or greater, and decimal points are omitted. Obeying Law and Rules and Taking Care are behavioural belief factors

Rules. Removing Time 1 behaviour reduced the variance explained to 47.6 per cent, a smaller decrement than in the Reasoned Action analysis (Figure 4.15).

Conclusion

The successful linking of social inputs at Time 1 to accident-related behaviour at Time 2, through path diagrams, was the culmination of a long and detailed series of analyses. The purpose of our investigation was to examine the effects of beliefs, perceptions and attitudes on behaviour and accident involvement, in a prospective design. The study was based on the Theory of Reasoned Action and the Health Belief Model, and strong links between beliefs and behaviour were found in both cases. By means of hierarchical modelling and path analysis we were able to show that beliefs and attitudes are best seen as mediators between inputs and outcomes. As much as 60 per cent of the variance in behaviour at Time 2 was explained,

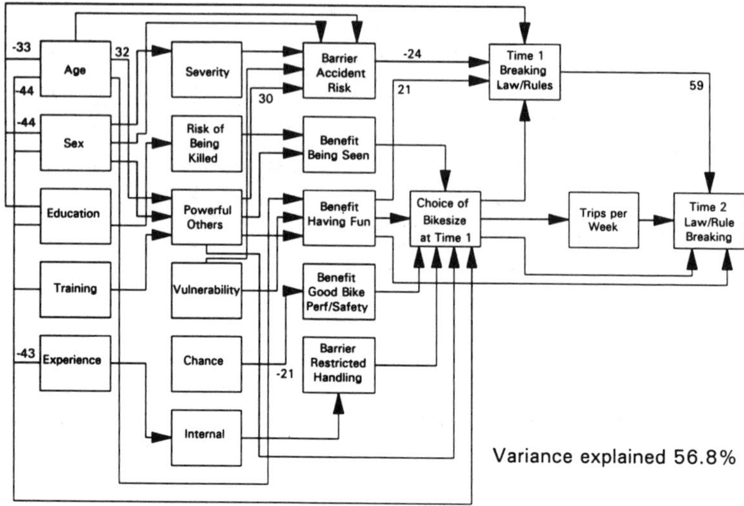

Figure 4.14 Health beliefs: path analysis for Time 2. Includes all variables with paths $p < 0.01$, but only those with betas 0.1 or greater are shown. Values are printed only for betas 0.2 or greater, and decimal points are omitted

considerably more than by any other approach to motorcycling safety we know.

Implications for theory, policy and practice

In this final section of the chapter we draw out the implications of our investigation for theory, and for policy and practice. The implications for theory concern the value of the Theory of Reasoned Action and the Health Belief Model for predicting safe and unsafe riding behaviours. The implications for policy and practice concern the value of the findings for informing future policy and practice in motorcycling safety.

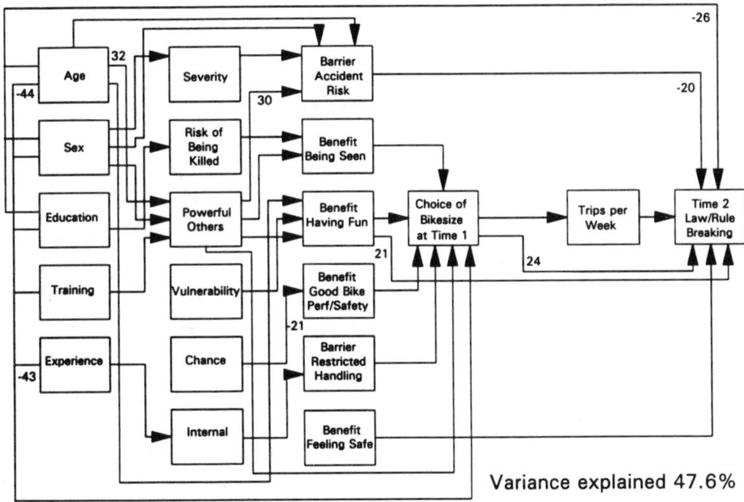

Figure 4.15 Health beliefs: Time 2 path analysis excluding prior behaviour. Includes all variables with paths $p < 0.01$, but only those with betas 0.1 or greater are shown. Values are printed only for betas 0.2 or greater, and decimal points are omitted

The value of psychological models for predicting road safety behaviour

The results show that both the Theory of Reasoned Action and the Health Belief Model can be used successfully to predict the frequency of riders' safe and unsafe riding behaviours. The main behavioural factor to predict accident involvement was 'Breaking Law and Rules', and we have shown that by measuring riders' beliefs and attitudes we were able to predict 40 per cent or 50 per cent of the variance in the factor twelve months later (38.4 per cent for the Theory of Reasoned Action and 47.6 per cent for the Health Belief Model). When behaviour at Time 1 was added to the prediction, the figure rose to over 60 per cent (63.3 per cent for the Theory of Reasoned Action and 62.0 per cent for the Health Belief Model).

That so much of the variance was explained has important

implications for understanding both road safety in general and motorcycling safety in particular. In the past, studies of motorcycling safety have often relied on either physical variables such as the type and colour of vehicles and equipment (for example, Thomson 1980; Olsen, Halstead-Nussloch and Sivak, 1981; Gilchrist, Mills and Khan, 1988) or biographical characteristics of the particular road-user group being studied (for example, Bragg, Dawson and Jonah, 1980; Bragg, 1981; Jonah, Dawson and Bragg, 1982; Koch, 1987). The significance of such variables, we have been able to show, is that they provide indirect measures of the underlying *psychological* determinants of road safety behaviour. For example, motorcycle engine size is an important predictor of unsafe riding behaviours – but is itself predicted by the beliefs and attributions of the rider. Engine size, we have argued, is therefore more usefully regarded for safety research as a measure of motorcycle 'choice' (a psychological variable) than a measure of the dimensions of the machine (a physical variable).

The 'variance explained' coin has a second side, of course, and that is that our analyses leave around half the variance in safe and unsafe riding behaviours *unexplained*. One of the assumptions at the beginning of our investigation was that motorcyclists along with pedal cyclists and pedestrians were 'vulnerable' rather than 'dangerous', in a way which neither they nor road users who 'threaten' them may appreciate. That motorcyclists whose beliefs were in favour of breaking the law and road safety rules were likely to ride more dangerously than other riders argues against our assumption. Similarly, Parker *et al.* (1992a, 1992b) in their work on car drivers have found that poor driving is marked less by errors and lapses than 'violations' (Reason *et al.*, 1990) – in which 'Breaking Law and Rules' would be included. What *does* support the notion of vulnerability, however, is that many riders with apparently 'good' beliefs and behaviour nevertheless reported accidents – as the variance we were unable to explain suggests. Research workers (for example, Nagayama, 1984; Brooks and Guppy, 1990) and our own respondents alike argue that the attitudes and behaviour of other road users towards motorcyclists will be an important area for future research. It is a view that we endorse.

Our investigation has shown that demographic variables such as age, sex, formal training and experience also play a role in safe and unsafe riding behaviours. Unlike physical measures such as engine size, however, they exert their influence *through* the rider's beliefs and attributions. In other words, the age, sex and experiences of a rider will influence his or her beliefs and attributions about motorcycling safety and it is these *psychological* variables that eventually determine the rider's choices and riding behaviour. Thus, psychological measures play a pivotal role in safe and unsafe riding behaviours, mediating between a rider's demographic characteristics and choice of vehicle and equipment.

In summary, the implications of our findings for theory in road safety research are threefold. First, psychological and social-psychological models of human behaviour contribute significantly to understanding accident liability among particular groups of road users by providing predictions of the safe and unsafe behaviours that determine accident liability. Second, an important source of variance in motorcycling accidents, as yet unexplored, is the attitudes and behaviours of other road users towards motorcyclists. Third, predictive statistical models of accident liability will prove most effective if they integrate demographic, physical and psychological variables within the broad framework of mediation described and tested in our research.

The value of the findings for future policy and practice

There are three main conclusions for policy and practice to be drawn from our findings. First, unsafe riding, as measured by law and rule breaking, is largely habitual in nature. However, the habit is underpinned by a complex structure of demographic and psychological determinants. Second, both the Theory of Reasoned Action and the Health Belief Model reaffirm the role of perceptions, attributions and beliefs as mediators between social inputs and behavioural outcomes, and it makes little difference which of the models is used. Third, we have been able to identify particular rider groups as being at greater risk of a serious road accident than the average rider, and we have begun to explore the practical implications, particularly for training.

The way in which high-risk groups are usually characterized –

by demographic variables such as age, sex and experience – tells us little about the underlying reasons for their high-risk status. Further analysis of our own data, however, has begun to identify the ways in which riders' demographic characteristics influence the safeness of their riding behaviour (Chesham, Rutter and Quine, 1990, 1991), and important implications are emerging for training. Intervention programmes, we believe, must be applied early in the motorcyclist's career before riding habits have been fully developed, and they must be designed to provide a cognitive underpinning for behaviour by instigating and developing beliefs and integrating them with behaviour. Both the Theory of Reasoned Action and the Health Belief Model are designed to inform programmes of attitude and belief change and are therefore well suited to providing a framework for safety training programmes.

It has long been acknowledged that formal motorcycling training does not necessarily improve the accident liability of riders, as we saw in the literature review early in the chapter. Research over the last decade has shown that formally trained riders are no safer than untrained riders, and indeed are sometimes less safe (Jonah and Dawson, 1979; Jonah, Dawson and Bragg, 1981, 1982; Mortimer, 1984, 1988; McDavid, Lohrmann and Lohrmann, 1989; Chesham, Rutter and Quine, 1990, 1991). As Mortimer comments: 'Those that had taken the course [the MSF motorcycle rider course] did not have a lower violation rate, a lower accident rate, a lower total cost of damage to accident-involved motorcycles, a significantly lower mean cost of injury treatment per accident, or a lower total cost of injury treatment. [However] those who had taken the course did have a lower mean cost of damage to the motorcycle per accident' (Mortimer, 1988, p. 187).

There have been many attempts to explain why training fails – based mainly on criticism of the content of existing programmes and the objectives behind them. Current training, we suggest, concentrates too much on developing the operating skills of trainees, and neglects the development of higher-order skills. As Jonah and Dawson concluded, after reporting that performance on the Motorcycle Operator Skill Test (MOST) did not predict subsequent accident involvement: 'It should be noted that lack of skill in riding a motorcycle may not be the only cause of motorcycle accidents and it may not even be the most important cause. Other factors such as the ability to perceive potentially hazardous situations and the willingness of motorcyclists to engage in risky riding behaviour could be more important than skill' (Jonah and Dawson, 1979, p. 164). That riders who are also car drivers have safer motorcycling records than other riders adds further support.

Training based on the findings of our own research would focus on improving the specific attributions, beliefs and attitudes identified as the most salient determinants of riding behaviour. If, for example, further analysis of the data were to reveal that the safeness of young motorcyclists' behaviour is largely determined by their perceptions of how 'powerful others' such as the police influence their accident involvement, then techniques to exploit the importance of normative influences would be applied. Clark and Powell (1984), for example, have shown that asking car drivers to make safety-related decisions *in groups* can be particularly effective, for normative influences become more apparent and salient in groups than when people are alone. Alternatively, if the safeness of young riders were found to depend more on their personal attitudes towards safety than on normative pressures, other techniques might prove more appropriate. Gregory, Borroughs and Ainslie (1985), for example, have had some success in changing people's attitudes towards traffic safety legislation by asking them to imagine 'self-relevant scenarios' of automobile accidents – scenarios where the person himself or herself is involved in an accident.

Other training techniques that may be useful for influencing the psychological determinants of safe and unsafe motorcycling include games and game-simulations (Mori and Peterson, 1986; Young and Lee, 1987; Renaud and Stolovitch, 1988), behavioural rehearsal (Jones *et al.*, 1989), and incentive schemes (Eddy, Marotto and Beltz, 1988). Each technique, however, is normally specific to only one psychological factor. Simulation, for example, focuses on improving hazard perception skills, while behavioural rehearsal focuses on improving the speed and efficiency of responses once the hazard has been perceived. It is important, therefore, to identify the most salient determinants of behaviour *before* one attempts to apply specific training techniques.

In summary, the implications of our findings for policy and practice are threefold. First, by relating the psychological determinants of safe and unsafe riding behaviours to the demographic characteristics of riders, we are able to identify high-risk groups according to their specific attributions, beliefs and attitudes. Second, psychological factors, unlike demographic factors such as age and sex, offer an opportunity for intervention. One cannot 'improve' the age and sex of an individual rider, but one can improve the attributions, beliefs and attitudes that provide the links between age and sex and the safeness of the rider's behaviour. Third, identifying the psychological determinants of safe and unsafe behaviour allows one to utilize more specialized and efficient techniques than at present for designing safety training programmes and mounting publicity campaigns.

References

Åberg L, Glad A, Bernhoft I M and Mäki M (1991), Social norms, attitudes and intentions concerning drinking and driving. A cross-national comparison, Unpublished, Uppsala University, Sweden.

Adams J G V (1981), *The Efficacy of Seat Belt Legislation*, London: UCL Department of Geography Occasional Paper 38.

Adams J G V (1987), Risk homeostasis and the purpose of safety regulation, *Ergonomics*, 31, 111–23.

Ajzen I (1988), *Attitudes, Personality and Behaviour*, Milton Keynes: Open University Press.

Allen H M and Taylor S E (1984), Alternative theories of health policy attitudes and protective behaviours: self-interest, sociotrophy and socialization, *Basic and Applied Social Psychology*, 5, 19–35.

Baker S P and Fisher R S (1977), Alcohol and motorcycle fatalities, *American Journal of Public Health*, 67, 246–9.

Bragg B W E (1981), Risk of accident involvement for motorcyclists. In *Road Safety*, Westport, CT: Praeger.

Bragg B W E, Dawson N F and Jonah B A (1980), Profile of the accident involved motorcyclist in Canada. In *Proceedings of International Motorcycle Safety Conference*, May 1980, Washington DC, 1131–51.

Brooks P and Guppy A (1990), The social context of driver error in accidents involving motorcycles: a theoretical framework and empirical exploration, *Driving Behaviour in a Social Context*, Caen: Paradigme, 1990.

Budd R J and Spencer C P (1986), Lay theories of behavioural intention: a source of response bias in the theory of reasoned action?, *British Journal of Social Psychology*, 25, 109–17.

Budd R J, North D and Spencer C (1984), Understanding seat belt use: a test of Bentler and Speckart's extension of the 'theory of reasoned action', *European Journal of Social Psychology*, 14, 69–78.

Cairns H (1941), Head injuries in motor-cyclists: the importance of the helmet, *British Medical Journal*, 2, 465–71.

Cairns H and Holbourn H (1943), Head injuries in motor-cyclists with special reference to crash helmets, *British Medical Journal*, 1, 591–98.

Chenier T C and Evans L (1987), Motorcyclist fatalities and the repeal of mandatory helmet wearing laws, *Accident Analysis and Prevention*, 19, 133–9.

Chesham D J, Rutter D R and Quine L (1990), Mapping the social psychological determinants of safe and unsafe motorcycling, *Transport and Road Research Laboratory/General Accident Symposium on Behavioural Research in Road Safety*, Nottingham, September.

Chesham D J, Rutter D R and Quine L (1991), Identifying the social-psychological determinants of safe and unsafe behaviour: the beliefs of male teenage motorcyclists. In M. Johnson, M. Herbert and T. Marteau (Eds.) *European Health Psychology*, Leicester: British Psychological Society.

Clark A W and Powell R J (1984), Changing drivers' attitudes through peer group decision, *Human Relations*, 37, 155–62.

Cohen J, Dearnaley E J and Hansel C E M (1958), The risk taken in driving under the influence of alcohol, *British Medical Journal*, June, 1438–42.

Colbourn C J (1978), Perceived risk as a determinant of driver behavior, *Accident Analysis and Prevention*, 10, 131–41.

Department of Transport (1991), *Road Accidents Great Britain 1990: The Casualty Report*, London: HMSO.

Eddy J M, Marotto D A and Beltz S M (1988), Analysis of a safety belt incentive program at CIGNA corporation, *American Journal of Health Promotion*, 2, 31–8.

Evans L (1985), Human behavior feedback and traffic safety, *Human Factors*, 27, 555–76.

Evans L (1991), *Traffic Safety and the Driver*, New York: Van Nostrand Reinhold.

Evans L and Wasielewski P (1981), Do accident-involved drivers exhibit riskier everyday driving behavior? *Accident Analysis and Prevention*, 13, 57–64.

Fishbein M and Ajzen I (1975), *Belief, Attitude, Intention and Behaviour*, Reading, Mass: Addison-Wesley.

Gielen A C, Ericksen M P, Daltoy L H and Rost K (1984), Factors associated with the use of child restraint devices, *Health Education Quarterly*, 11, 195–206.

Gilchrist A, Mills N J and Khan T (1988), Survey of head, helmet and headform sizes related to motorcycle helmet design, *Ergonomics*, 31, 1395–412.

Graham J D and Lee Y (1986), Behavioral response to safety legislation: the case of motorcycle helmet-wearing legislation, *Policy Sciences*, 19, 253–73.

Gregory W L, Borroughs W J and Ainslie F M (1985), Self-relevant scenarios as attitude change, *Personality and Social Psychology Bulletin*, 11, 435–44.

Hobbs C, Galer I and Stroud P (1983), *Attitudes, Opinions and Knowledge of Motorcyclists*, Loughborough: Loughborough University of Technology.

Janz N K and Becker M H (1984), The health belief model: a decade later, *Health Education Quarterly*, 11, 1–47.

Jonah B A and Dawson N E (1979), Validation of the motorcycle operator skill test, *Accident Analysis and Prevention*, 11, 163–71.

Jonah B A, Dawson N E and Bragg B W E (1981), Predicting accident involvement with the motorcycle operator skill test, *Accident Analysis and Prevention*, 13, 307–18.

Jonah B A, Dawson N E and Bragg B W E (1982), Are formally trained motorcyclists safer? *Accident Analysis and Prevention*, 14, 247–55.

Jones H V and Heimstra N W (1964), Ability of drivers to make critical passing judgments, *Journal of Engineering Psychology*, 3, 117–22.

Jones R T, Ollendick T H, McLaughlin K J and Williams C E (1989), Elaborative and behavioral rehearsal in the acquisition of fire emergency skills and the reduction of fear of fire, *Behavior Therapy*, 20, 93–101.

King J B (1982), The impact of patients' perceptions of high blood pressure on attendance at screening: an extension of the health belief model, *Social Science and Medicine*, 16, 1079–91.

Knoflacher H (1974), Accident risk for passenger cars and single track two wheeled motor vehicles (translation), *Straßenverkeherstechnik*, Heft 6.

Koch H (1987), The correlation between and the influence of age, riding experience and engine performance on the involvement of motorcycle beginners in accidents: results of multivariate evaluations of a survey. Paper presented to joint conference of VDI (Association of German Engineers) and BMW: *Active and Passive Safety of Motorcycles*.

Kraus J F, Franti C E, Johnson S L and Riggins R S (1976), Trends in deaths due to motorcycle crashes and risk factors in injury collisions, *Accident Analysis and Prevention*, 8, 247–55.

Kraus J F, Riggins R S and Franti C E (1975a), Some epidemiological features of motorcycle collision injuries – I. Introduction, methods and factors associated with incidence, *American Journal of Epidemiology*, 102, 74–98.

Kraus J F, Riggins R S and Franti C E (1975b), Some epidemiological features of motorcycle collision injuries – II. Factors associated with severity of injuries, *American Journal of Epidemiology*, 102, 99–109.

Kristiansen C M (1987), Social learning theory and preventive health behaviour: some neglected variables, *Social Behaviour*, 2, 73–86.

Langer E J (1978), Rethinking the role of thought in social interaction. In J H Harvey, W Ickes and R F Kidd (Eds.) *New Directions in Attribution Research*, Vol. 2, Hillsdale, NJ: Lawrence Erlbaum.

Langlie J K (1977), Social networks, health beliefs and preventive health behaviour, *Journal of Health and Social Behavior*, 18, 244–60.

Leaman A and Fitch M (1986), Perception of risk in motor-cyclists, *Archives of Emergency Medicine*, 3, 199–201.

McDavid J C, Lohrmann B A and Lohrmann G (1989), Does motorcycle training reduce accidents? Evidence from a longitudinal quasi-experimental study, *Journal of Safety Research*, 20, 61–72.

Mori L and Peterson L (1986), Training pre-schoolers in home safety skills to prevent inadvertent injury, *Journal of Clinical and Child Psychology*, 15, 106–14.

Mortimer R G (1984), Evaluation of the motorcycle rider course, *Accident Analysis and Prevention*, 16, 63–71.

Mortimer R G (1988), A further evaluation of the motorcycle rider course, *Journal of Safety Research*, 19, 187–96.

Motorcycle Safety Foundation (1979), *Motorcycle Helmet Use: Behavioral Aspects*, MSF Research Department, USA.

Nagayama Y (1984), An analysis of accidents involving motorcycles and suggestions for drivers' education, *IATSS Research Report*, 8, 28–39.

National Highway Traffic Safety Administration (USA) (1980), *The Effect of Motorcycle Helmet Use Repeal – A Case for Helmet Use*, Publication No. US–DOT HS–805–312.

Nelson G D and Moffit P B (1988), Safety belt promotion: theory and practice, *Accident Analysis and Prevention*, 20, 27–38.

Newman J A (1976), Characteristics of motorcycle accidents, *Proceedings of the Meeting on Biomechanics of Injury to Pedestrians, Cyclists and Motorcyclists*, Amsterdam: International Research Committee on the Biokinetics of Impact.

Office of Population Censuses and Surveys (1991), *Mortality Statistics 1989: Cause*, London: HMSO.

Olsen P L, Halstead-Nussloch R and Sivak M (1981), The effect of improvements in motorcycle/motorcyclist conspicuity on driver behavior, *Human Factors*, 23, 237–48.

Parker D, Manstead A S R, Stradling S G and Reason J T (1992a), Determinants of intention to commit driving violations, *Accident Analysis and Prevention*, 24, 117–31.

Parker D, Manstead A S R, Stradling S G, Reason J T and Baxter J S (1992b), Intention to commit driving violations: an application of the Theory of Planned Behavior, *Journal of Applied Psychology*, 77, 94–101.

Prem H and Good M C (1984), *Motorcycle Skills Assessment*, Melbourne: Australian Office of Road Safety.

Raeder P K and Negri D B (1969), *An Evaluation of Motor Vehicle Accidents Involving Motorcycles*, Research Report of the New York State Department of Motor Vehicles, New York.

Reason J, Manstead A, Stradling S, Baxter J and Campbell K (1990), Errors and violations on the roads: a real distinction?, *Ergonomics*, 33, 1315–32.

Renaud L and Stolovitch H (1988), Simulation gaming: an effective strategy for creating appropriate traffic safety behaviors in five-year-old children, *Simulation and Games*, 19, 328–45.

Robertson L S (1976), An instance of effective legal regulation: motorcyclist helmet and daytime headlamp laws, *Law and Society Review*, 10, 468–77.

Rotter J B (1966), Generalized expectancies for internal versus external control of reinforcement, *Psychological Monographs*, 80 (Whole No. 609).

Rutter D R, Quine L and Chesham D J (1990), Do motorcyclists' beliefs predict accident liability? In T. Benjamin (Ed.) *Driving Behaviour in a Social Context*, Paris: La Routière.

Rutter D R, Quine L and Chesham D J (1992), Behavioural health models: predicting safe riding in motorcyclists. In J A M Winnubst and S Maes (Eds.) *Lifestyles, Stress and Health*, Leiden: DSWO Press.

Simpson C H (1983), Motorcycle press exposure study, *Transportation Research Record*, 909, 30–9.

Stasson M and Fishbein M (1990), The relation between perceived risk and preventive action: a within-subject analysis of perceived driving risk and intentions to wear seatbelts, *Journal of Applied Social Psychology*, 20, 1541–57.

Stradling S (1990), Police sanctions in changing driver behaviour, *Driving Behaviour in a Social Context*, Caen: Paradigme.

Sutton S and Hallett R (1989), Understanding seat-belt intentions and behavior: a decision-making approach, *Journal of Applied Social Psychology*, 19, 1310–25.

Thomson G A (1980), The role frontal motorcycle conspicuity has in road accidents, *Accident Analysis and Prevention*, 12, 165–78.

Vaughan R G (1976), A study of motorcycle crashes, Paper to the

Motorcycles and Safety Symposium, Australian Road Research Centre, Melbourne, Australia, June.

Watson G S, Zador P L and Wilks A (1981), Helmet use, helmet use laws and motorcyclist fatalities, *American Journal of Public Health*, 71, 297–300.

Webb G R, Sanson-Fisher R W and Bowman J A (1988), Psychosocial factors related to parental restraint of pre-school children in motor vehicles, *Accident Analysis and Prevention*, 20, 97–4.

Wilde G J S (1982a), The theory of risk homeostasis: implications for safety and health, *Risk Analysis*, 2, 209–25.

Wilde G J S (1982b), Critical issues in risk homeostasis theory, *Risk Analysis*, 2, 249–58.

Wilde G J S (1985), Assumptions necessary and unnecessary to risk homeostasis, *Ergonomics*, 28, 1531–8.

Williams A F, Ginsberg M J and Burchman P F (1979), Motorcycle helmet use in relation to legal requirements, *Accident Analysis and Prevention*, 11, 271–3.

Wittenbraker J, Gibbs B L and Kahle L R (1983), Seat belt attitudes, habits, and behaviors: an adaptive amendment to the Fishbein model, *Journal of Applied Social Psychology*, 13, 406–21.

Young D S and Lee D N (1987), Training children in road-crossing skills using a road side simulation, *Accident Analysis and Prevention*, 19, 327–41.

Chapter 5

Discussion and Conclusions

We come now to the final chapter of the book. From the outset, our purpose has been clear: to identify the ways in which social psychological variables affect health outcome and, in particular, how they mediate the influence of social inputs upon outcomes. Social inputs are the variables that have traditionally concerned epidemiologists – sex, age, social class, and so on – and our goal has been to explore the causal pathways from inputs through social psychological mediators to outcomes.

To guide our research we began by developing a theoretical model. The model identifies two sets of social psychological variables, which we believe link inputs to outcomes: socio-emotional variables and cognitive variables. The principal socio-emotional variables we have considered are people's experiences of severe life-events and difficulties, and the availability and adequacy of supportive relationships offering cognitive guidance, tangible assistance, emotional support, social reinforcement and opportunities for social interaction. People's experience of severe life-events and the social support they have are determined in part by social inputs such as social class, age, marital status and education. The experience of severe life-events, in combination with low social support, we argue, leads to emotional problems, including loss of self-esteem, anxiety and depression. The main cognitive variables we have examined are people's access to information, their knowledge and their cognitive dispositions. Poor education results in less knowledge and in poverty of access to information which, in turn, we believe, affect cognitive dispositions. Cognitive dispositions include personal control, beliefs and attitudes, all of which we see as products of information, knowledge and communication.

At the heart of our model lies coping. Coping is about the ways in which people confront the stresses in their lives, and we argue that the resources and strategies available to them – and the way they select and implement them – are products of both the socio-emotional and cognitive levels of our model. For example, people who lack social support and are already weakened by adversity may have fewer coping strategies to call upon than people who are free from adversity and have access to supportive relationships – and the strategies they select may differ too. Again, people with optimistic explanatory styles, who focus on external, unstable and specific explanations for life's difficulties, may display different coping patterns from people with pessimistic styles, who expect bad events to occur consistently and uncontrollably, and who react with helplessness, depression and passivity. Socio-emotional and cognitive problems may act separately or in combination, and they result in coping styles and strategies characterized by helplessness or hopelessness, altered perceptions of risk and vulnerability, and an undue willingness to behave in risky ways. From dysfunctional coping styles come inappropriate behaviours, and from inappropriate behaviours come negative health outcomes.

The three central chapters of the book presented our own empirical research – on pregnancy outcome, breast cancer and motorcycling. In each case, key inputs and outcomes were identified from the epidemiological literature, and an attempt was made to explore the significance of social psychological mediators. In the case of pregnancy, which we discussed in Chapter 2, the main social input we identified was social class, which is known to be of great importance both for 'hard' outcomes such as pregnancy complications, morbidity, low birthweight and mortality, and for 'soft' outcomes such as satisfaction – with maternity care, with the birth experience and with medical communications at the time of the birth. We reported three studies from our programme of research. The first examined parents' satisfaction with maternity care, and drew attention to the importance of pre-existing attitudes and knowledge and their links with social class. The second examined women's satisfaction with the quality of their birth experience, and pointed to the significance of social class and age as inputs and social support and information as mediators. The third study examined doctor–parent communication, in the context of breaking the news of severe mental impairment, and again social class was shown to be an important input. Of the social psychological mediators, socio-emotional aspects of the doctor's behaviour proved to be far more important for satisfaction with communication than did the cognitive or information content of what was said.

In Chapter 3 we turned to breast cancer screening. The epidemiological evidence shows that age, social class, marriage and motherhood are all significant predictors of outcome – where outcome refers to incidence, survival and mortality. The most important mediator between inputs and outcomes is early diagnosis – but the only way at present to achieve early diagnosis over the population as a whole is to ensure that women attend for regular X-ray mammography. The key issue for social psychological research, we therefore argued, was who does and does not attend for screening. The prediction of attendance and non-attendance provided the focus for the first part of our own research, and we were able to show that social psychological factors played a leading role. Among the most important were the woman's attitude to screening, how strongly she believed her family and friends wanted her to attend, and whether she thought circumstances would permit her to attend. In the second part of our programme we examined the process of mammography itself, particularly the extent and nature of discomfort and pain. Three main findings emerged: the discomfort of screening was generally less than women expected and less than the discomfort of other medical interventions, including cervical screening and giving a blood sample; it was greatest in women who expected that the procedures would be painful; and only rarely did it lead women to say that they would turn down future invitations to screening.

In Chapter 4, the last of our empirical chapters, we reported our research on motorcycling safety. It is well established in the official statistics that the most likely riders to have accidents are young men. The relationship is very strong – among the strongest of all the input–outcome relationships we have identified in the book – yet hardly anything is known about the links, let alone the detailed patterns of mediation. Using our model to set up a variety of possible pathways, we were able to show that accidents were associated with particular patterns of behaviour – notably willingness to break the laws and rules of safe riding – and that behaviour was in turn predicted by perceptions of control and by attitudes. Social inputs and accident outcomes were thus *mediated* by behaviour and by social psychological 'risk factors'. The pattern of relationships was among the clearest we have found in all our research, and the findings offered good support for our model.

In the remainder of the chapter, we turn now to the further implications of our model and findings. Throughout the book, our concerns have been with theory, and with policy and practice. Our purpose now is to draw together the arguments we have set out, and we begin with theory.

Theoretical issues

Conceptual questions

The concept of mediation

The first conceptual issue to discuss is the theoretical utility of the concept of mediation. Throughout the book, our main tenet has been that social psychological variables are best seen as mediators between social inputs and health outcomes. We have seen our task as twofold: to explore which variables are important for which areas of health; and to draw out the possible links. The question we must confront now is what does our approach offer that traditional approaches do not – where traditional approaches confine themselves to epidemiology or to social psychology, but pay little attention to the links between them.

There are three main answers. First, through our model we are able to provide at least some of the mechanisms and processes that 'explain' the facts that epidemiology has revealed. For example, infant mortality is greater in working-class families than in middle-class families, and we have been able to suggest at least part of the answer to the question why: the link is *mediated*, through life-events, social support, cognitive dispositions, coping and behaviour. Again, as we have seen, young male motorcyclists have higher accident rates than other motorcyclists, and mediation helps to explain the relationship once more: this time, locus of control, cognitive dispositions and behaviour are the most important social psychological variables.

The second answer is that our approach is able to *quantify* the patterns of mediation, by means of path analysis. That is, we are able to *weight* the relative importance of the mediating variables and to test their strengths statistically. The third answer, which leads on from the second, is that we are able to test when effects are direct and when they are indirect. For example, we knew from the previous literature that middle-class women are generally less satisfied than working-class women with breast screening, but we did not know whether the path was direct or indirect. By using the framework provided by our model we were able to show that the path was indirect, through discomfort: middle-class women experienced more discomfort than working-class women, and it was discomfort that made them less satisfied. For epidemiology our approach is thus able to 'explain' some of the bald epidemiological facts; and for social psychology, it puts familiar mechanisms into an epidemiological context and gives them a central role in explaining health outcomes – which without the links back to epidemiological social inputs they would be denied.

The components of our model

The second of our conceptual issues is how well can the various components we have built into our model be distinguished. There are really two questions: first, are concepts we regard as distinct actually distinct; and second, have we assigned the concepts to their correct levels or groups in the model? An example of the first problem is provided by the history of the concept of attitude. Until the late 1960s, attitude was a composite term, that encompassed – or, more accurately, confounded – three dimensions: cognition, affect and conation. The literature was moribund but then, as we have seen, a turning point came, for the dimensions were separated, by Fishbein and Ajzen, into belief, attitude and intention (Fishbein and Ajzen, 1975). Theoretical interest in attitudes quickly revived, and the literature has developed rapidly ever since because conceptually the separation made sense, and empirically it was supported too. Our own model similarly will be refined as the concepts it incorporates change and develop, and we hope it too may encourage new growth in the literature.

The second question, whether we have assigned the concepts to their appropriate levels and groups in our model, is more difficult to answer. A good example this time is Type A Behaviour Pattern. The name itself suggests that the variable is a behaviour, but sometimes it is seen as a coping mechanism, often it is regarded as a basic personality trait, and we have chosen to place it in a group of variables labelled 'personal control'. Conceptually, it may be possible to justify any or all of those choices, and the only way to reach a solution will be by *empirical* testing. How best to regard a variable conceptually must sometimes be determined by where in one's theoretical structure it adds most to the statistical power of the analysis.

Testing and developing the model

The final set of conceptual issues concerns the future, and there are two main questions to address. The first is about the best strategy to adopt for testing the model, whether 'micro' or 'macro'. The micro or 'bottom-up' approach to mediation takes one set of variables at a time – input, mediator and outcome – and attempts to join the various sets later. The macro or 'top-down' approach offers a putative model of all the mechanisms of interest and attempts to test all the relationships at once. For practical reasons the micro approach is easier, of course, and has generally been preferred. Thus, for example, there are enormous literatures on the roles of locus of control, coping and behaviour in mediating class and health, but because of the micro approach the literatures are more than enormous: they are separate. The time has therefore come, we believe, for a move towards macro strategies, for it is the *overall* pattern of relationships that matters most. Only through top-down analyses will it be possible to determine the causal ordering of variables, their relative weights (both individually and in groups), and whether genuine mediation can be demonstrated.

This last issue, testing for the occurrence of genuine mediation, is particularly important. Although conceptually the causal pathways we have suggested may make sense, many have yet to be confirmed statistically. As Baron and Kenny (1986) point out, mediation is best tested by conducting three regression analyses: first, the mediator is regressed on the independent variable; second, the dependent variable is regressed on the independent variable; and third, the dependent variable is regressed on both the independent variable and the mediator. If mediation *is* present, three conditions will hold: the independent variable will affect the mediator in the first analysis; the independent variable will affect the dependent variable in the second analysis; and the mediator will affect the dependent variable in the third analysis. If all three conditions hold in the predicted direction, the effect of the independent variable on the dependent variable must be less in the third analysis than in the second. Full analyses of the sort that Baron and Kenny suggest have as yet seldom been conducted, and they will need extensive data collection and the continued application of sophisticated techniques of multivariate statistical analysis.

If the first issue for the future of our model is how best to test it, the second concerns its limitations. The model we have outlined is intended as a framework for integrating past findings and for guiding future research. We do not wish to suggest that all links between social inputs and health outcomes are mediated in the way the model emphasizes. There may well, for example, be direct links between some of the inputs and some of the outcomes, or indirect links through behaviour that bypass social psychological mechanisms altogether. Moreover, we acknowledge that the model is oversimplified, not least in that all the causal pathways we include are seen as left to right with no allowance for feedback loops. In fact, feedback loops are likely to be of great importance. For example, it may be that reducing how much one smokes affects not only health outcomes but also variables that occur earlier in the model – such as perceived locus of control and attitudes. Changes in those variables may in turn encourage a further reduction in smoking, so that outcomes are improved still more. To take another example, improved coping may feed back to social support, so that people who begin to cope better make new friends, which helps them to cope better still. Detailed statistical analysis of descriptive data and controlled intervention through experimental approaches will both be necessary to establish the role of feedback, and a careful consideration of how best to design future studies will be needed.

Design questions

Prospective designs

One of the difficulties for social psychologists is how to assess the relative importance of the plethora of studies that appear to show possible causal relationships between social psychological factors and health outcomes. In the literature on social support, for example, there are many studies that show a relationship between low social support and psychiatric illness. Many, however, have been retrospective – psychiatrically ill people were asked to recall their social networks before the onset of the illness – or cross-sectional – measures of current social support and illness were taken at one point in time. Associations demonstrated in these ways are open to a number of interpretations: depressed people may have a gloomy view of their social networks; their symptoms may put people off; or personality traits may lead both to the development of depressive symptoms and to the inability to form and maintain relationships. If proper evidence of a causal relationship is to be demonstrated, the straightforward requirement is to conduct prospective longitudinal studies. Prospective studies identify and follow up a group of subjects, collecting data at a number of points in time. Their essential feature is that measures of the 'independent variable' are taken before the 'dependent variable' happens, so that the dependent variable can be properly predicted, in advance.

Suppose for a moment that we have carried out a prospective study, and our observations reveal a clear-cut relationship between two variables. What aspects of the association should be considered before deciding that the most likely explanation is a causal one? Simon (1978) argues that the demonstration of causality involves three distinct operations: the first is demonstrating covariance; the second is eliminating spurious relationships; and the third is establishing the time order of the occurrences. Demonstrating covariance simply means that two or more phenomena vary together. Showing that the observed covariation is non-spurious involves demonstrating that the relationship between the variables cannot be explained by a third variable. Establishing the time order of the variables requires the researcher to demonstrate that one phenomenon occurs first or changes before another phenomenon. Where we are trying to make links between disease or health outcomes and aspects of the environment, a number of considerations must be taken into account. One of the classic papers on the subject, by Hill (1965), proposes eight criteria to be considered when inferring causality: strength, consistency, specificity of outcome, temporality, biological gradient, biological plausibility, coherence and experimental intervention. Though Hill argues that none is a hard-and-fast rule that must be obeyed before we accept cause and effect, the criteria are important and we shall explore them in more detail. Their value is in helping us to decide whether there is any way of explaining the set of facts before us other than by cause and effect.

The first criterion specified by Hill is strength: what is the size of the effect? In a famous early example, the London surgeon Pott was able in 1775 to implicate the occupation of chimney sweeping in scrotal cancer – by comparing the occupations of patients with scrotal cancer with the occupations of patients presenting with other diseases, and finding a marked excess. In another classic analysis, this time of the opening weeks of the cholera epidemic of 1854, John Snow (1855) was able to deduce the cause by recording a death rate of 71 per 10,000 houses of customers supplied with the polluted water of the Southwark and Vauxhall company, compared with a rate 14 times lower of 5 per 10,000 supplied with sewage-free water. Through Snow's analysis, a way of preventing cholera was thus discovered thirty years before the water-borne organism responsible for the disease was isolated. A more modern example is the work of Doll and Peto (1976), who showed that the death rate from cancer of the lung in cigarette smokers is 10 times the rate in non-smokers, and the rate in heavy smokers is over 20 times the rate in non-smokers.

When so strong a relationship is discovered, Hill's first criterion has been more than met, and there are good grounds for suspecting cause and effect.

Hill's second criterion is consistency: has the association been observed repeatedly by different people in different places, circumstances and times? For example, the Advisory Committee to the Surgeon-General of the United States Public Health Service found an association between smoking and cancer of the lung in 29 retrospective and 7 prospective inquiries (US Department of Health, Education and Welfare, 1964). Without such consistency, there would have been little reason to pursue cause and effect any further.

The third criterion is the specificity of the association: is the association between specific variables or between classes of variable? If, for example, the association is limited to a specific occupation, and to particular sites and types of disease, and there is no association between the occupation and deaths from other diseases, there is a clear argument in favour of a causal link. To take another example, if a variety of causes of death are raised 10 or 20 per cent in smokers, but death from lung cancer is raised by 900 per cent, there is greater specificity for lung cancer than for the other diseases and therefore greater reason to suspect cause and effect there than elsewhere.

The fourth of Hill's criteria is the temporal relationship of the association: for example, do severe life-events cause depression or do depressed people report more severe life-events? The essential requirement is to date the event accurately, particularly in relation to the time of onset of symptoms: the event must precede the onset of illness in order for a causal argument to be sustained.

The fifth of Hill's criteria is biological gradient: is there a gradient relating 'dose' to outcome? If the association is one that can conceivably reveal such a gradient, then the evidence should be carefully sought. An example where a biological gradient *is* likely is the association between smoking and lung cancer, for the death rate rises linearly with the number of cigarettes smoked daily allowing us to hypothesize a cause-and-effect relationship. Other examples are the dangers of dust in industry, or pollution in the environment: the more dust and pollution, the greater the incidence of disease that can be expected.

The sixth criterion is biological plausibility: is cause and effect theoretically possible given the current state of medical knowledge? Hill notes that what is biologically plausible depends on the knowledge of the day, and the association may be one that is quite new to medical science. He reminds us of Sherlock Holmes' advice to Dr Watson: 'When you have eliminated the impossible, whatever remains, however improbable, must be the truth.' Despite this exhortation, Hill emphasizes in his seventh criterion that the cause-and-effect interpretation of data should not seriously conflict with the generally known facts of the natural history and biology of disease. It should have *coherence*.

The eighth and last criterion that Hill proposes is the effect of experimental intervention: does intervention produce a change in outcome? Suppose, for example, that the dust in a factory is reduced, or people stop smoking cigarettes or reduce their intake of fat. Is the frequency of the associated events affected? Hill argues that experimental or quasi-experimental evidence will often be the strongest test of cause–effect hypotheses.

Experimental designs

The classic experimental or intervention design includes two comparable groups: an experimental group and a control group. The two groups are equivalent, except that the experimental group is exposed to the independent variable and the control group is not. Membership of the two groups is determined by random assignment. Imagine, for example, that we are interested in whether the provision of social support will prevent a high-risk group of patients who have been exposed to severe life-events becoming depressed. To assess the effect of the independent variable (social support) we would take measurements of the dependent variable (symptoms of illness) from each group after the experimental group had received the intervention. If the symptom score for the experimental group is significantly lower than for the control group, it is inferred that the independent variable is causally related to the dependent variable. Such a design is often referred to as a non-treatment control group design, and variations include placebo control designs, where patients are assigned to treatment or placebo treatment control groups. In research into the efficacy of drugs, for example, the placebo control design often takes the form of a double-blind trial, in which an experimental group of patients receiving an active drug are compared with a control group receiving an identical but pharmacologically inert placebo. Both the patients and the administering personnel are ignorant of the nature of the pills taken by any one person.

The essence of experimental designs is intervention, and a classic example again comes from John Snow. Snow (1855) noted several features of the cholera outbreak in mid-nineteenth-century London: the disease began with alimentary tract symptoms; people who shared a room with someone who had died did not necessarily contract it; and cases were distributed widely over quite large areas rather than affecting everyone within a local district. When in 1849 a severe outbreak occurred in central London, Snow tested his theory that cholera was related to contaminated drinking water by removing the handle of the pump in Broad Street from which most of the people who had died obtained their drinking water. The outbreak subsided.

A more recent example of a successful intervention comes from Oakley, Rajan and Grant (1990), who conducted a randomized controlled study of the effect of social support on pregnancy outcome for women with histories of low-birthweight babies. 'Intervention' babies were on average 38 g heavier than 'control' babies; fewer were born with very low birthweights; and spontaneous onset of labour and spontaneous vaginal delivery were both more common in the intervention group.

A further example, from our own work, is women's expectations of pain during breast cancer screening, reported in Chapter 3. Women who expected screening to be painful were more likely to report discomfort than women who had no such expectations. Most women, moreover, reported that the discomfort of screening was less than they had expected, and less than for other medical procedures: having a tooth drilled, having a cervical smear test and giving a blood sample. The implication is that an intervention study to encourage positive expectations, by offering accurate and representative information about discomfort and pain to women about to attend screening, would have an important part to play in reducing discomfort.

Issues for policy and practice

Defining and setting objectives

Policy and practice are about strategy and tactics: defining and setting objectives; planning how to implement them; and doing the implementation itself. Determining policy and setting objectives are the preserve of politicians, not social psychologists. However, social psychologists have a role to play in initiating and advising on plans to implement a given set of objectives. It is here, we believe, that our approach, which links social inputs through social psychological mediators to outcomes, has much to offer. Before we can begin to outline the contribution we believe our approach makes, we need to examine what politicians consider to be the goals we need to be working towards. In Chapter 1, we saw that the World Health Organization in 1978 set out what it called a 'Global Strategy for Health for All by the Year 2000'. Twelve objectives were defined for the international community, and the onus was on individual governments to develop coherent health policies, with proper strategies and plans of action, to try to reach those objectives. The principal route, urged WHO, should be through primary care.

In Britain – or strictly England – the Government's current policy was first set out in a consultative document published in 1991, called *The Health of the Nation* (Department of Health, 1991). Responsibility for health, the document argued, lay with local health authorities, and their task was threefold:

> first, to assess the state of health of the people they serve; second, to obtain the services needed to ensure effective action is taken to maintain good health, prevent and treat ill-health, rehabilitate people to good health, and provide support and care for those who are disabled, chronically ill or dying; third, to ensure the quality and effectiveness – including cost effectiveness – of the services their residents use.

Nationally, the Government's strategy would be to identify for attention key areas where improvements could be made; within those areas, to place the emphasis on securing genuine improvements in health for which targets could be set at either national or local level and progress monitored; and to seek to improve knowledge and understanding in order to review and reappraise priorities over time and bring further areas within the scope of national priorities and targets. The criteria for selecting the areas for special attention would be: that the area should be a major cause of premature death or avoidable ill-health (sickness and/or disability) either in the population as a whole or among specific groups of people; that it should be an area where effective interventions were possible, offering significant scope for improvement in health; and that it should be possible to set objectives and targets in the particular area and monitor progress by means of indicators.

At the heart of the consultative document lay the objectives and targets the Government named as priorities. There were sixteen key areas. After consultation, a revised version of the document was published as a White Paper in July 1992: *The Health of the Nation: A Strategy for Health in England* (Department of Health, 1992). The key areas had now been grouped, and there were five, each with a brief statement of the Government's objectives and a set of associated measurable targets. The five areas were coronary heart disease and stroke, cancer, mental illness, HIV/AIDS and sexual health, and accidents.

For the first area, coronary heart disease and stroke, the Government's objective was apparently simple: to reduce the level of ill-health and death caused by coronary heart disease and stroke, and the risk factors associated with them. Together, coronary heart disease and stroke are responsible for almost 40 per cent of all deaths in this country, and the majority of the targets were concerned with what, in the Government's view, were among the leading causes of the problem: smoking, diet, and drinking. There were nine specific targets.

1. To reduce death rates for both coronary heart disease and stroke in people under 65 by at least 40 per cent by the year 2000.
2. To reduce the death rate for coronary heart disease in people aged 65–74 by at least 30 per cent by the year 2000.
3. To reduce the death rate for stroke in people aged 65–74 by at least 40 per cent by the year 2000.
4. To reduce the prevalence of cigarette smoking in men and

women aged 16 and over to no more than 20 per cent by the year 2000.

5. To reduce the average percentage of food energy derived by the population from saturated fatty acids by at least 30 per cent by 2005.
6. To reduce the average percentage of food energy derived by the population from total fat by at least 12 per cent by 2005.
7. To reduce the percentage of men and women aged 16–64 who are obese by at least 25 per cent for men and at least 33 per cent for women by 2005.
8. To reduce mean systolic blood pressure in the adult population by at least 5 mm Hg.
9. To reduce the proportion of men drinking more than 21 units of alcohol per week from 28 per cent in 1990 to 18 per cent by 2005, and the proportion of women drinking more than 14 units of alcohol per week from 11 per cent in 1990 to 7 per cent by 2005.

After coronary heart disease, the next most common cause of death in England is cancer – 25 per cent of deaths in 1991. Cancer was the second priority area for the Government, and there were three principal objectives: to reduce ill-health and death caused by breast and cervical cancer; to reduce ill-health and death caused by skin cancers – by increasing awareness of the need to avoid excessive skin exposure to ultra-violet light; and to reduce ill-health and death caused by lung cancer – and other conditions associated with tobacco use – by reducing smoking prevalence and tobacco consumption throughout the population. For the first of those objectives there were two main targets: (1) to reduce the death rate for breast cancer in the population invited for screening by at least 25 per cent by the year 2000; and (2) to reduce the incidence of invasive cervical cancer by at least 20 per cent by the year 2000. For the second objective, there was just one target: to halt the year on year increase in the incidence of skin cancer by 2005. For the third objective, there were five targets: (1) To reduce the death rate for lung cancer by at least 30 per cent in men under 75 and 15 per cent in women under 75 by 2010. (2) To reduce the prevalence of cigarette smoking in men and women aged 16 and over to no more than 20 per cent by the year 2000. (3) To ensure that, in addition to the overall reduction in prevalence, at least a third of women smokers should stop smoking at the start of their pregnancy by the year 2000. (4) To reduce the consumption of cigarettes by at least 40 per cent by the year 2000 (from almost 100 billion manufactured cigarettes in 1990). (5) To reduce smoking prevalence among 11–15 year olds by at least 33 per cent by 1994.

The third of the Government's areas was mental health. Mental illness is a leading cause of ill-health and disability. It accounts for about 14 per cent of certificated sickness absence, 14 per cent of NHS in-patient costs, and 23 per cent of NHS pharmaceutical costs. The objective stated in the White Paper was simply 'to reduce ill-health and death caused by mental illness'. There were three main targets: (1) to improve significantly the health and social functioning of mentally ill people; (2) to reduce the overall suicide rate by at least 15 per cent by the year 2000; and (3) to reduce the suicide rate of severely mentally ill people by at least 33 per cent by the year 2000.

The fourth area was HIV/AIDS and sexual health, and this time there were six objectives: (1) to reduce the incidence of HIV infection; (2) to reduce the incidence of other sexually transmitted diseases; (3) to develop further and strengthen monitoring and surveillance; (4) to provide effective services for diagnosis and treatment of HIV and other sexually transmitted diseases; (5) to reduce the number of unwanted pregnancies; and (6) to ensure the provision of effective family planning services for people who want them. There were three specific targets: (a) To reduce the incidence of gonorrhoea among men and women aged 15–64 by at least 20 per cent by 1995. (b) To reduce the rate of conceptions amongst the under 16s by at least 50 per cent by the year 2000 (from almost 10 per 1,000 girls aged 13–15 in 1989). (c) To reduce the percentage of drug users who report sharing needles in the previous four weeks by at least 50 per cent by 1997, and by at least a further 50 per cent by the year 2000.

The final area was accidents, and here the objective was simply to 'reduce ill-health, disability and death caused by accidents'. There were three targets: (1) To reduce the death rate for accidents among children aged under 15 by at least 33 per cent by 2005. (2) To reduce the death rate for accidents among young people aged 15–24 by at least 25 per cent by 2005. (3) To reduce the death rate for accidents among people aged 65 and over by at least 33 per cent by 2005. All types of accident – home, work, roads, and so on – were treated as one.

The Government's statement is important because it has set the agenda for the foreseeable future. Each objective is concerned with what we have called outcomes, and the targets are measurable so that effectiveness can be monitored. The choice of priorities is a matter of debate, of course, as also are the precise targets – why sometimes the year 2005, for example, rather than 2000 – but the White Paper is nevertheless an important attempt to focus attention on goals and achievement. The question now is how are the objectives to be achieved, and it is here, we believe, that our analysis of health outcome has a part to play.

Meeting objectives

Among the most coherent commentators on the original consultative document was the *British Medical Journal*, the journal of the British Medical Association, the 'governing body' of British doctors. In *The Health of the Nation: the BMJ View* (Smith, 1991), each of the original sixteen priority areas was discussed in turn, and five questions were asked about each one: should it be a key area; was there a case against; what should the targets be for each one; what should be the strategy for reaching those targets; and what were the barriers? That the sixteen areas were eventually presented as five groups in the White Paper was in part attributable to the influence of the BMA's response. Much was also made by the BMA of what it perceived as weaknesses in the Government's strategy for meeting its objectives and targets, and again noticeable changes were made by the time the White Paper was published. As the editor of the *BMJ* book wrote: 'The easy part of strategic planning is devising a strategy. The difficult part is making it happen' (Smith, 1991, p. 5).

The approach to 'making it happen' that the Government takes in its White Paper varies greatly across the five key areas, but a number of themes recur. Indeed, they are often implied by what are seen as the key objectives and targets in the first place. First, there is an emphasis on individuals' behaviour. For example, smoking, diet and drinking are seen as important contributors to coronary heart disease and stroke – smoking is emphasized again in cancer – and the Government believes that people must be made to change. Second, the view of the White Paper is that change will come about through 'dissemination of information' and 'encouraging and enabling changes' to be made. Third, the responsibility for dissemination and encouragement is seen as belonging to a variety of key agencies: the Health Education Authority, the National Health Service, local authorities, the voluntary sector, the caring professions, the media, manufacturers (of cigarettes and alcohol, for example) and employers. Fourth, the Government sees a large part of its role as co-ordinating those agencies, and setting standards, enacting and enforcing legislation, providing guidance and allocating resources.

The White Paper has been a significant attempt to identify priorities for health outcomes, to set objectives and targets, and to begin to offer strategies for reaching those objectives and targets. From our own viewpoint, however, it fails in two major respects: it pays little attention to social structural variables in health; and it says almost nothing about how, in practice, strategies for change are to be turned into workable everyday procedures. In both respects, our own approach has a contribution to make.

Implications of our model

The central purpose of our model has been to draw attention to the role of social structural variables in health outcomes, and to the mechanisms by which they have their effects. The overwhelming priority for policy-makers, we believe, must be to confront the effects of social structural variables directly. An important part of our argument is demonstrated by what is known about social deprivation. In Chapter 1, we discussed the Black Report, which demonstrated that people at the bottom of the social scale were twice as much at risk of almost every form of morbidity and mortality as people at the top. The Black Report was published in 1980, since when the social divide has become wider still (Whitehead, 1987). Deprivation has direct effects on health –

leaking roofs cause bronchial illness – but there are indirect effects too. Poverty may restrict diet, for example, which produces ill-health; and, even further back in our model, poor education in deprived populations may lead to inadequate knowledge about prevention, for example, and so to misunderstanding about the value of health screening, and thus to a reluctance to take up screening services. In each case, whether directly, indirectly through behaviour, or indirectly through knowledge and so behaviour, the starting point is social inputs, and it is those that must be addressed above all.

An important part of the problem is the provision of services. In the last of our examples, take-up of screening, the emphasis of the White Paper is on the behaviour of the individual: the service is there to be used, but the individual 'fails' to take up the invitation, and it is therefore the individual that must be changed. We shall return to behaviour in a moment, but there is of course much more, for what superficially may appear to be inappropriate behaviour may in fact be the result of defects in the service. The National Breast Screening Programme provides a useful example. Until the late 1980s there *was* no national service. Then, many years after similar programmes had been set up in other countries in Europe, the first dedicated screening centres were funded. But there were many inadequacies: centres were often inaccessible, and women in deprived areas could simply not reach them; publicity and information were initially poor so that women did not know or understand what was on offer; staff training for what was to be a specialized and sensitive occupation was often brief and hasty; and little attention was paid to quality assurance. Even today, in our own research, we have seen that an important source of dissatisfaction is undue delay in receiving the result. If services are not designed and funded properly, tailored to the client population (Robson, Boomla and Savage, 1986), and evaluated continually, they will not be taken up. It is to the failure of the service, not only the apparent failure of individual behaviour, that policy must be directed.

Changing people's behaviour, in our view, is best seen as *part of* providing proper services, and not an objective in itself or an alternative to structural change. What matters most about behaviour within the framework of our model is what underpins it, for only by analyzing and understanding the underpinnings of behaviour can we begin to plan how best to change it. Three examples will illustrate what we mean. First, in research on pregnancy outcome, Oakley was able to show that women who lacked social support were at special risk (Oakley, Rajan and Grant, 1990). The mechanisms linking social support to outcome were unclear – though our model suggests that the effects of socio-emotional and cognitive variables on behaviour are likely to have been central – but measurable benefits were found when the women were given extra visits and help from midwives. No attempt had been made to change behaviour directly, but manipulating the key variables that *underpinned* behaviour produced significant effects.

Our second example comes from smoking. Many attempts have been made to induce smokers to give up by direct behavioural intervention (Hunt and Bespalec, 1974; Bernstein and McAlister, 1976; Fagerstrom, 1984). Our own model suggests a quite different approach: first, we must understand the processes that lead people to take up smoking in the first place; and second, we must make sense of the mechanisms by which they sustain and maintain the behaviour. We have seen that social inputs are strongly implicated in the decision to start smoking, and that life-events, social support, locus of control and particular coping styles underpin the maintenance of the behaviour. Quite different approaches will be needed for the two problems – perhaps structural change for the former, and an emphasis on socio-emotional and cognitive mechanisms for the latter – and again our model suggests where to start and what are likely to be the most successful theoretical and practical approaches. As always, theory remains the first requirement.

Our final example comes from our own research on motorcycling safety. As we have seen, young men are the most likely riders to have accidents. By using our model and the statistical procedures associated with it, we have been able to show that youth is more important than the lack of experience that normally goes with it, and that the principal mediator of the behaviours that lead to accidents is cognitive structure. That is, young male riders often do not understand *why* they should ride in particular ways and take particular precautions, and so they do not. Accidents follow. The solution we have suggested is to modify training, so that the emphasis is moved away from what to do to why to do it. We must understand the social inputs that lead to health outcomes; we must identify the social psychological mediators that link inputs to outcomes, and trace the causal pathways; and we must build policy and practice on the findings that emerge. That has been the argument at the heart of our book.

References

Baron R M and Kenny D A (1986), The moderator–mediator variable distinction in social psychological research: conceptual, strategic, and statistical considerations, *Journal of Personality and Social Psychology*, 51, 1173–82.

Bernstein D A and McAlister A L (1976), The modification of smoking behaviour, *Addictive Behaviour*, 1, 89–102.

Department of Health (1991), *The Health of the Nation: A Consultative Document for Health in England*, London: HMSO.

Department of Health (1992), *The Health of the Nation: A Strategy for Health in England*, London: HMSO.

Doll R and Peto R (1976), Mortality in relation to smoking: 20 years' observations on male British doctors, *British Medical Journal*, 2, 1525–36.

Fagerstrom K O (1984), Effective nicotine chewing gum and follow up appointments in physician-based smoking cessation, *Preventive Medicine*, 13, 517–27.

Fishbein M and Ajzen I (1975), *Belief, Attitude, Intention and Behavior*, Reading, Mass: Addison-Wesley.

Hill A B (1965), The environment and disease: association or causation?, *Proceedings of the Royal Society of Medicine*, 58, 295–300.

Hunt W A and Bespalec D A (1974), An evaluation of current methods of modifying smoking behaviour, *Journal of Clinical Psychology*, 30, 431–8.

Oakley A, Rajan L and Grant A (1990), Social support and pregnancy outcome, *British Journal of Obstetrics and Gynaecology*, 97, 155–62.

Robson J, Boomla K and Savage W (1986), Reducing delay in booking for antenatal care, *Journal of the Royal College of General Practitioners*, 36, 274–5.

Simon J (1978), *Basic Research Methods in Social Science*, 2nd edition, New York: Random House.

Smith R (Ed.) (1991), *The Health of the Nation: The BMJ View*, London: *British Medical Journal*.

Snow J (1855), *On the Mode of Communications of Cholera*, 2nd edition, London: Hafner.

US Department of Health, Education and Welfare (1964), *Smoking and Health*, Public Health Service Publications No. 1103, Washington.

Whitehead M (1987), *The Health Divide: Inequalities in Health in the 1980's*, London: Health Education Council.

Index